THE 5 PILLARS WICCA

 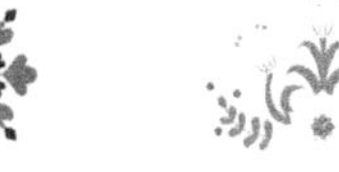   

FOUNDATIONS **BELIEFS** **PRACTICE** **MAGICK** **RITUALS**

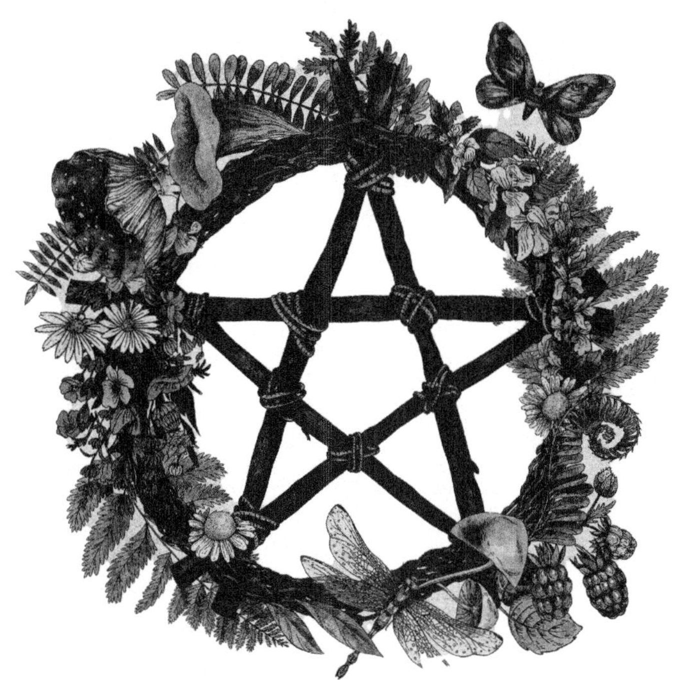

115 TECHNIQUES & TIPS

to Connect to Your Higher Self with the Magick and Rituals of Witchcraft. Find Inner Balance and Harmony by Harnessing the Power and Wisdom of the Craft

INGRID CLARKE

Table of Contents

Introduction

When you hear the word "Wicca," what image does it conjure up in your mind? Likely, your vision of Wicca and its practices could be different from another person's. But this does not mean you are wrong. Wicca is varied and multifaceted, making it a practice and lifestyle with which people from numerous backgrounds can adopt and grow a connection. There are countless ways to understand and experience Wicca's essence. And different people may practice it uniquely, which is perfectly fine. Despite the different approaches to Wicca, the basic tenet of interconnectedness remains unchanged.

Wicca brings harmony and balance to one's life, which, during troubling times, is essential. And as inherently spiritual, it raised introspection and questioning how to better connect with oneself and the world. Practicing Wicca helps bring the connection back into your life, whether with the earth, yourself, or others.

This book distills the spiritual principles and practices of the craft that can open your awareness, connect you to the divinity of the world you are living in, and awaken the magick in you. In this book, I will break down the different aspects of Wicca through the five pillars: foundation, beliefs, practice, magick, and rituals. These pillars help shape how we understand and interact with the world.

Daily life contains stress, anxiety, and other negative aspects. These stresses might be caused by work, issues you are facing in your relationship, or troubles you are having with your personal life. In today's modern world, it is becoming easier and easier to detach from our natural environment and ourselves. As we become accustomed to this detachment, it becomes harder to understand our inner natures.

Having suffered severe burnout, my family's Scandinavian roots in neo-paganism drove me to look into different healing techniques. Through my research, I was able to accumulate many teachings and wisdom. Subsequently, I did not only study Wicca but also many metaphysical practices and occult traditions from around the world. And by my exploration and practice, I realized that I was an empath. Now, my mission in life is to share my extensive knowledge and experiences with those who need help and healing. This book will serve as an introduction to Wicca and its practices. The first two pillars will increase your knowledge of Wicca, including its history and modern-day significance, as well as describe its core beliefs and principles. Meanwhile, pillars three to five will talk about Wiccans' different techniques, rituals, ways of worship, and magickal practices.

Throughout this book, we will discuss multiple strategies to help you better understand and align yourself with the elemental nature of the universe. You will find 115 beginner techniques, tips, and strategies to awaken the magick within you and forge a deep connection with your higher self. It's peppered throughout the entire book and it's intentionally designed this way to serve as your guide along each step of the process. I have practiced all the methods discussed in this book, which have empowered me to find ways through any challenges and provided me with a means for self-development and positive change. It is essential to remember that the only way to enact changes in your life is to take charge, and the techniques you will learn in this chapter will enable you to do so. The end goal of this book is to help you with your journey of spiritual awakening and help you to get in touch with your higher self and find your divine purpose. By tapping into your intuition, Wicca offers a path for stirring up celestial magick within yourself. And with this book, you will gain a blueprint for activating the power of divine magick and opening yourself up to its wonders.

Despite the challenges in gaining knowledge about Wicca and its practices, this book makes it accessible for anyone interested in uncovering its mysteries. Regardless of the struggles you are dealing with in your life, the timeless wisdom of the craft will provide a different point of view on how to approach life's complexities. Alongside this awareness, you will uncover inspiration, beauty, and revelations as you rewrite your destiny and uncover the mysteries of the unknown. With proper usage of what you will learn here, you can create a new place for yourself and comprehend the enigma. Hence, by the end of this book, you will have begun your self-discovery journey; all that remains is to access divine power within yourself.

Accordingly, each chapter of this book will give you a better understanding of Wiccan beliefs and conventions, as well as steps and strategies for those looking to walk the Wiccan path and create better connections with their inner self, others, and the world. Likewise, this book will teach you how to open your mind to possibilities and enhance your life. Now, let us dive into the first pillar of Wicca and learn about its foundation.

Pillar 1
Foundations

Wicca is an ancient religion practiced for thousands of years and can be traced back to old Pagan traditions. Today, it is a modern neo-Pagan spirituality based on honoring the natural world, respecting all life forms, and finding the balance between the dark and light to reach a divine understanding. Pillar 1 seeks to explain Wicca and how it has evolved throughout history so you can make more informed decisions when exploring this path.

1

What is Wicca?

Before we can get into the fundamentals or traditions of Wicca, let us take a step back and look at what it is. Subsequently, Wicca is the largest neo-Pagan religion, also called modern Pagans, with followers known as Wiccans, who typically identify themselves as witches. Before the 1950s, Wiccans kept their practices hidden— only coming to light in England and other Western countries. Anyhow, their followership is a few hundred thousand individuals. And although there are no direct ties to Christianity, Wicca was highly influenced by European religions. Now that you have a fundamental definition of Wicca let us dive into the old religion, history, and the prevalence of Wicca in the modern day.

Old Religion

Many religions throughout history have had figures known as witches, some of whom were evil figures, and in others, they were healing and good creatures. There is a long history of old religions that, although not responsible for the creation of the Wiccan religion, is connected to it because Wiccans associated themselves with witchcraft and called themselves witches. Christianity has a long history with witches, although it is seldom a positive one.

The general ideals around witchcraft and witches have changed during the modern day, with it being used in films as a trope of good and evil and a means of resolving social tensions, especially in feminism. However, pre-modern Western civilization held a lot of irrational fear around witchcraft. This fear often stemmed from religious practices claiming witchcraft was the devil's work. Inevitably, the fear sired a hostile mentality towards those identified as witches.

From there, witch hunts started in the 11th century and continued into the 18th century. With the propagation of witchcraft as heresy and devil's work by Christianity and other religions resulted in those accused receiving persecution. As fear continued to grow and fester around the ideas of witches, by the 14th century, it was commonly believed that all people that were witches used a form of malevolent sorcery and were evil.

Witches continued to be regarded with trepidation and linked to the devil. Even the meaning of their rituals, such as the sabbats, was twisted, and it was believed that they gathered to perform orgies and other sexual acts in the name of Satan. It also became a belief that they could transform, had familiars, and kidnapped and murdered children. Think back to the tale of "Hansel and Gretel." It was written long before the creation of Wicca and portrayed a witch that would lure children in and eat them. Although these are ideas of fantasy, they stuck so much fear into people that laws were created to punish those that were witches and allowed for witch hunts to occur. Notably, witch hunts were rarely about capturing those already regarded as 'witches.' But instead, it focused on tracking down those suspected to be hiding.

The Salem Witch Trials also showed religious intolerance, fear, and political control, with numerous women accused of witchcraft being hanged. Altogether, these trials led to the execution of 19 individuals of all ages. However, there was no proof that these people were witches, but rather it is theorized that family feuds, religion, politics, and fear were the cause of the accusations and executions. One person accusing another of their bad fortune was enough to raise suspicion about them being witches. People's fear of witches became so ingrained in the culture that indictments and prosecutions occurred in villages, law courts, and courts of Appeal in Protestant and Roman Catholic communities. Studies have shown that approximately 110,000 people were on record of being tried as witches, and about 40,000 to 60,000 of these trials resulted in executions.

Law and religion played equal parts in witch trials and hunts, and over the years, cultures developed numerous ways to determine whether someone was a witch. The first way was to prick them. If they felt no pain, they were a witch, as the devil had desensitized them to it. A devil's mark, often an oddly shaped mole, was also looked for. Meanwhile, some throw people into lakes and ponds.

Interestingly, it was believed that if an accused person sunk in the water during a trial by ordeal, it was indicative of their innocence as the water was seen to be accepting them; witches would not prevail. These signs were mainly used in local and village trials, while more extensive trials, such as those held before kings, inquisitors, and bishops, resulted in fewer convictions and milder sentences. This is likely due to a heavier influence on the law than religion, although both still played a part in both trials.

Witchcraft and witches have also been linked back to ancient civilizations, as it was believed that magick and religion were needed to appease, manipulate, and protect against evil spirits. These civilizations thought that evil spirits were universal, so magick was necessary. It could also be used for evil at the time. Sabbats have often been compared to the rituals performed in the worship of Dionysus, as people would gather outside and perform many rituals, including sacrificing animals, feasting, drinking, and orgies.

History and Origin

The origins of Wicca can be traced back to a British civil servant by the name of Gerald Brosseau Gardner. He spent most of his career traveling throughout Asia, and during his time there, he learned about many indigenous religions and traditions. He also invested much of his time reading the writings of British occultist Aleister Crowley and other esoteric literature.

Gardner returned to England in the 1930s and joined a British occult community, which claimed they had located a group of witches near New Forest in 1939. Gardner claims that he and the occult group communicated with the New Forest group of witches, and the information they learned from them was the basis on which Wicca was formed. In 1951, the archaic witchcraft laws were repealed, which enabled Gardner to form his coven, publish *Witchcraft Today*, and create the Gardnerian Wicca religion with Doreen Valiente, who served as a high priestess.

Gardner formed not all Wiccan practices, beliefs, and rituals; instead, he helped to jumpstart other occultists to develop their Wiccan traditions throughout the 1950s and '60s.

Most Wiccans claimed they were practicing pre-Christian witchcraft. However, historians disputed this as more studies of modern witchcraft continued. In the 1960s, Wicca emerged as a general term for religion, yet, there were various forms, including Alexandrian. During the first two decades, most Wiccans were initiated into covens, but as time continued, more and more people initiated themselves into Wicca. Many forms of Wicca were created during its emergence, which we will discuss later in this book. The beauty of Wicca comes from the varied ways you can practice it.

Wicca in the Present

Although Wicca was never at the scale of Christianity in terms of followers, it gained popularity throughout America and western culture. Numerous books started to be published in the 1970s and '80s, telling people how they could initiate themselves into Wicca. Although covens are few and far between in the present day, individual Wiccans are still practicing. It is unknown how many people are still actively practicing Wicca, as many initiated themselves and practice solitarily rather than in a coven. In the present day, Wicca, or witchcraft, is more known as a trope in film, television, and books than as a religion.

As Wicca was traveling through America as a religion, it also grabbed the public eye as it became the subject of many films and television series, including *Buffy the Vampire Slayer*, *Charmed*, and *The Craft*. However, many of the portrayals of Wiccans in popular media have caused people to fear those who practice Wicca or have gone on to create false tropes and representations of its ideals. Teenage Wiccan culture was heavily portrayed in the media, often warning young teenagers of the dangers of practicing, which has resulted in a decrease in initiates over the years. Because of the negative portrayals of the Wiccans in mainstream media, many tried to rebrand themselves as traditional witches, but this insinuated that they partook in non-Wiccan occultism and rituals.

Wicca and witchcraft, over time, have started to become used interchangeably. However, it is important to note the difference. Witchcraft has been connected to many religions throughout history, but Wicca has only existed for less than 100 years. Wicca is said to be derived from witch practices; the name Wicca is etymologically connected to the word witch, which is why followers call themselves witches. Yet, this is not concrete proof that the New Forest witches were accurate, which many historians have tried to prove and disprove.

Now that you know the foundations of Wicca, its history, and it in the modern day, it is time to move on to the second pillar and learn all about the beliefs of the Wiccans. Remember that there might be some variation between the different types of Wicca in terms of faith. Still, they all stem from spiritual empowerment and connecting with oneself and the world around you. The first aspect of Wiccan beliefs that we will discuss is deities.

Pillar 2
Beliefs

There is power in understanding, and with learning comes growth. Now, we will explore the tenets of Pillar 2 about Wiccan's beliefs. And through understanding its various components, we can form a more meaningful connection to this ancient spiritual practice.

In Chapter 2, we will learn about the Horned God and the Moon or Triple Goddess. Meanwhile, Chapter 3 will teach us about the five elements: earth, air, fire, water, and spirit or aethyr. Next, Chapter 4 will explain the Wiccan rede, a code of morals for Wiccans.

Then we will move on to Chapter 5, covering both greater and lesser Sabbats, which include religious holidays like Samhain and Yule and seasonal phenomenons such as Spring Equinox and Summer Solstice. And finally, Chapter 6 reveals rituals surrounding birth (wiccaning), marriage (handfasting), separation (hand-parting), death (crossing the bridge), and afterlife/reincarnation.

We have much to learn before us on our journey into the deep wisdom of this sacred practice; let us begin!

2
Deities

Undoubtedly, the gods and goddesses worshiped in Wicca are among the prominent declarations of faith for devotees of this religion. Unlike Christianity, which only worships one god or deity, Wicca is similar to Ancient Greece or Rome, as there are two central deities. However, the ancient Greeks, Romans, and other cultures worshiped many different gods as they served as symbols for various reasons, such as the harvest, youth, changing of seasons, and fertility, amongst many other things. Whilst Wicca and neo-Paganism have two central deities— the Horned God and the Triple Goddess. In this chapter, we will discuss the origins of each of these deities and their purpose within Wicca.

The Horned/Sun God

Although the Horned God has become tightly linked to Wiccan practices and neo-Paganism, the name was first used in the early 20th century to describe anthropomorphic gods that took on the image of antlered or horned animals. And looking throughout history, many religious beliefs have incorporated horned deities.

The word "witch" is typically believed to be feminine, while "warlock" is masculine. Yet, within the context of Wicca, the distinction between a witch and a warlock has no gender implications. In truth, some followers of witchcraft chose to refer to themselves as witches regardless of gender since warlock was seen as a derogatory word. Nevertheless, the Horned God in Wicca represents the masculine side of Wicca. Likewise, Wicca is known as a duotheistic theology system, which means that masculine and feminine are equal within the system, and both are needed. Depictions of the Horned God differ depending on the source. Some sources show him as having horns or antlers, while the rest of him is human. Other depictions will show him as having an animal head and a human body, thus representing the union between the divine and animals. In this instance, the animal is often a representation of humanity.

Wiccan beliefs also associate the Horned God with the life cycle, nature, hunting, the wilderness, and sexuality. He is also considered a dualistic god, representing two aspects of something: day and night, light and dark, and summer and winter, along with others. As he is associated with the life cycle, his duality can also be connected to life and death.

The Horned God is the consort of the Triple Goddess, but they are both equals within the religion. He is considered masculine, and she the feminine. Often, they serve to represent opposites. Wiccans, like other religions, tend to organize the world in terms of masculine and feminine energy. Anything masculine, such as hunting and the wilderness, is associated with the Horned God.

Although Wiccan believed that the gods and goddesses were both equally important, recent developments have seen a far greater emphasis on the feminist influences of the Goddess, a reflection of feminism's growing mark. Meanwhile, the Horned God is a fundamental part of Wicca worshippers' Wheel of the Year celebrations, symbolizing the cycle of seasons. During the year, he is said to impregnate the Triple Goddess during the spring, die as winter approaches, and is then reborn by the Goddess with the new year.

Aside from that, the Horned God is often compared to Hades, the Greek God of the underworld, as they reside over hell. The Horned God was also Summerland's protector, the realm in which souls awaited reincarnation. Remarkably, the death of the Horned God in the Wheel of the Year resembles Persephone's story, where she stayed in the underworld with Hades before her triumphant return as a harbinger of spring. Unlike other religions, the Horned God's relation to death does not cause fear within followers; instead, he is considered a comforter and consoler to those who have passed and are waiting to be reincarnated.

Moon/Triple Goddess

Wicca is not the only neo-Paganism religion that is practiced. In many of them, the Triple Goddess is a deity, or at least a deity archetype in the religion's practices. The Triple Goddess is often referred to as a Moon Goddess, but her representation as a triunity, a combination of three figures, is the most common. These representations tied to the Triple Goddess include the female life cycle (the maiden, the mother, and the crone), three realms of the world (heaven, earth, and underworld), and the phases of the moon, hence why she is often referred to as a Moon Goddess. Yet, Wicca did not create this figure like the Horned God. While most commonly associated with Wicca, the Triple Goddess has a long religious history extending beyond its modern context.

The origins of a Triple Goddess started during ancient history, including ancient Greece with the Graces, the Horae, and the Moirai. It is also connected to the Hindu religion with the representation of Tridevi. The goddess Hecate, in ancient Greece, was thought to be one of the first Triple Goddesses due to her presence in art and sculptures during her early worship. Later, the Roman goddess Diana, also known as Artemis in Greek mythology, was depicted as a Triple Goddess. Yet, Hecate is significant for the Triple Goddess in Wicca because she associates with witchcraft.

Likewise, she was heavily connected to the moon, and her triple nature was seen to be related to the moon's phases.

Within Wicca, the physical female body is viewed as sacred since it reflects the Triple Goddess, a representation of femininity associated with birth, lactation, menstruation, and female sexuality. This depiction of the Triple Goddess as different areas of a woman's life includes the following distinctions:

- The maiden or child represents birth, new possibilities, youthfulness, inception, and expansion. The maiden is described as a waxing moon if there are connections to the moon.
- The mother represents fulfillment, fertility, sexuality, ripeness, power, and life. This stage is often depicted as the full moon, which could symbolize pregnancy.
- The crone or older woman represents repose, wisdom, endings, and death. This stage is defined as a waning moon.

During the 1970s, The Triple Goddess had a special significance for female followers when feminist movements blossomed. Her image brought solace and liberation to many who sought her out. Although she had a consort, The Triple Goddess was often solitary in the days following his death, a role that transcended what was traditionally viewed as masculine. Thus, she was transformed into an image of self-sufficiency and encouraged Wiccan women to take on more traditionally male roles, especially as more and more coven leaders were becoming women rather than men.

Wicca draws influence from the Horned God and the Triple Goddess, with their combined power representing the five-pointed pentacle symbol. The Horned God is known for his duality, while the Triple Goddess manifests threes; together, they give form to the powerful five-pointed star. Their meaning and how you worship them differ depending on the type of Wicca one is practicing. Still, no matter how you practice Wicca, these two deities are critical for spiritual empowerment and learning to connect with oneself. For female Wiccans, the Triple Goddess is paramount because she is an influential figure they look up to and can connect with at all times. In the next chapter, we will explore the importance of the elements in Wiccan beliefs.

3
Elements

For Wiccans, magick is simple and effective. It is not complicated or convoluted but rather is a part of nature. Thus, when someone can connect with their spirituality and the world around them, they should be able to use the elements as a form of magick. Primarily, Wiccans embrace the foundational elements of air, fire, earth, and water with an extra fifth element, spirit or aether, for their metaphysical practice. This blend of both physical and spiritual components brings their magick to life. And this chapter will explore how each element is vital to Wiccan beliefs and rituals.

Spirit or Aether

Before we talk about the four traditional elements, we must first talk about the influence spirit or aether has on one's ability to perform elemental magick and its effect on a person. One's energy or spirit is essential for performing magick. In Wicca, spells and words are only used to guide focus; the person's spirit performs that magick. One's spirit can also play a large part in influencing the elements. When someone has a light or good spirit, their effect on the elements will be positive, while someone with a dark or negative soul will have a negative impact. For example, with earth, someone who has a good spirit can help the land and even produce gems. But someone with a bad spirit will cause earthquakes and damage. Spirit and energy are present within each of the four other elements, which enables Wiccans to influence them.

Air

Wiccans are deeply connected to air, the first masculine element, and associated with the Horned God and his practices. This warm and moist element is symbolic of spring. Although air is intangible, it is seen as a powerful element more influential than tangible substances like water and earth. During rituals involving air, wands and staffs symbolize this element, and incense and smudge sticks are used as part of the ceremony. These air spells are typically connected to healing or purification.

Fire

Fire is considered one of the most spiritual elements and is on the masculine spectrum. Although it has no physical form like water or earth, it creates warmth and light and is believed to have powerful transformative abilities. Likewise, it is a warm and dry element associated with summer. Candles are one of the most commonly used tools for fire magick, along with burning spells and rituals. Meanwhile, red and gold gems, such as red jasper, tiger's eye, rubies, and bloodstones, are used in fire magick along with herbs and spices, such as allspice and cinnamon. Lastly, fire magick is associated with power, creativity, strength, love, and passion.

Earth

Earth has strong ties to the goddess, making it a common element used in the practices of Wicca. Salt, onyx, and aventurine are often used within these rituals to draw upon the prosperity and abundance associated with earth magick. This is mainly due to its connection with the Triple Goddess and the earth's fertility. Yet, not only does earth bring about life and new beginnings, but also death and rebirth. When we die, we return to the earth; our decomposition sustains new generations of life. Lastly, winter months are connected to earth as an element as they can be described as cold and dry.

Water

Water is another feminine element and is considered superior as it has more motion and activity than the element of earth, which is known for being sturdy and stable. This is why it is one of the most prominent magick in Wicca. But what makes it unique is its ability to interact with our senses. Associated with fall, this cold, moist element closely connects emotions, water's undulating waves are often likened to tears shed in both times of sorrow and joy, symbolizing the deep emotional currents it embodies. Symbols like water lilies or aloe plants, alongside gems like amethyst, aquamarine, and opal, are often integrated into this magick.

The Elements and Spiritual Direction

The elements are not only used for elemental magick, but according to Selena Fox, a high priestess of the Circle Sanctuary coven, they also serve as a "framework of spiritual symbology, teachings, and practices" (*Wicca manual, n.d.*) that Wiccans have. Elements are a framework, as each element is associated with different sacred directions. The rituals you practice can differ depending on which element you are influenced by the most. People can also have times when they are more connected to one element over others. However, the majority of Wiccans try to connect with all five elements. Here are each of the directions that the elements are associated with:

- Earth is associated with the north.
- Air is associated with the east.
- Fire is associated with the south.
- Water is associated with the west.
- Spirit is associated with the center because each human holds their spirit.

The pentacle is a symbol that represents Wiccans' ability to bring spirit to the earth or the elements. The five elements are often placed on the pentacle as a way of showing how each of the elements is essential for different areas of one's life, and unity of all five is needed for spiritual empowerment and wholeness. Here are how the elements are arranged on the pentacle and which areas of one's life they influence:

- Earth influences physical endurance and stability and is placed on the lower left corner of the pentacle.
- Fire influences daringness and courage and is placed in the lower right corner of the pentacle.
- Water influences intuition and emotions and is placed on the upper right of the pentacle.
- Air influences thoughts, intelligence, and the arts and is placed on the upper left of the pentacle.
- Spirit is placed on the top point of the pentacle and represents oneself and the divine.

People who are physically active and fit will likely be more connected to the earth than the other elements.

The elements play a large part in Wiccan beliefs and practices. Wicca enables people to connect with themselves and nature, understanding the importance of the elements in our lives and acknowledging the damage or healing we can do to nature. In the next chapter, we will start to dive deeper into Wiccan beliefs as we explore their ethics and the Wiccan rede.

4

Ethics

As with any religion, there are ethics that followers must identify with. Typically, the ethics associated with a religion is what draws people in. Although there are different ways to practice Wicca, those doing it for good all follow the same moral codes outlined in the Wiccan Rede and the Rule of Three. In this chapter, we will explore the Wiccan Rede, the Rule of Three, and their importance to Wiccan ethics and beliefs.

The Wiccan Rede

The Wiccan Rede is essential to the beliefs and practices of the Wiccans. It outlines the moral standards associated with Wiccans and other neo-Paganism religions. The word rede is derived from the words advice and counsel. Wiccans often seek out the Wiccan Rede during hard times. It is believed that the first iteration of the Wiccan Rede was publicly recorded by Doreen Valiente in 1964. The first form of the Wiccan Rede was only composed of eight words which varied in different forms. The original Wiccan Rede read: "An ye harm none, do what ye will" (*Wiccan rede*, 2022).

In 1974, a longer Wiccan Rede, which would become the one officially recognized, was published and is as follows:

Bide the Wiccan Laws, we must In Perfect Love and Perfect Trust.
Live and let live. Fairly take and fairly give.
Cast the Circle thrice about to keep the evil spirits out.
To bind the spell every time, let the spell be spake in rhyme.
Soft of eye and light of touch, speak little, listen much.
Deosil goes by the waxing moon, chanting out the Witches' Rune.
Widdershins go by the waning moon, chanting out the baneful rune.
When the Lady's moon is new, kiss the hand to her, times two.
When the moon rides at her peak, your heart's desire seeks.
Heed the North wind's mighty gale, locked the door,
and dropped the sail.
When the wind comes from the South, love
will kiss thee on the mouth.
When the wind blows from the West,
departed souls will have no rest.
When the wind blows from the East, expect the new and set the feast.
Nine woods in the cauldron go, burn them fast and burn them slow.
Elder be the Lady's tree, burn it not, or cursed you'll be.
When the Wheel begins to turn, let the Beltane fires burn.
When the Wheel has turned to Yule,
light the log, and the Horned One rules.
Heed ye flower, Bush and Tree, by the Lady, blessed be.
Where the rippling waters go, cast a stone, and truth you'll know.
When ye have a true need, hearken not to others' greed.
With a fool, no season spend, lest ye be counted as his friend.
Merry meet and merry part, bright the cheeks and warm the heart.
Mind the Threefold Law, you should,
three times bad and three times good.
When misfortune is enow, wear the blue star on thy brow.
True in love ever be, lest thy lover's false to thee.
Eight words the Wiccan Rede fulfill: An ye harm none, do what ye will. (*The Wiccan Rede, n.d.*)

The Wiccan Rede is much like all religions' fundamental Golden Rule. The majority of Wiccans, no matter which type, follow the Wiccan Rede. However, a small group of Gardnerian Wicca chooses to use the Charge of the Goddess, specifically the following line as their moral code: "Keep pure your highest ideal, strive ever toward it; let naught stop you or turn you aside, for mine is the secret door which opens upon the door of youth" (*Wiccan rede,* 2022).

The Charge of the Goddess is fundamental to all Wiccans and their practices; however, it typically is not used as a moral code. This poem is used during many rituals. During that time, the priest or priestess leading the ceremony became a representation of the Triple Goddess. The Charge describes how the Triple Goddess will guide and teach the Wiccans. It is essential to their practice and beliefs, despite the Wiccan Rede being the standard moral code.

There is often debate around the meaning of the Rede, with some Wiccans believing it to be a commandment, while others believe it to be advice. There is no statement of what precisely the Wiccans Rede means, and it is left to the individual's interpretation of what to make of it. The common understanding is that the Wiccan Rede tells followers to do good for others and themselves. Another interpretation of the Wiccan Rede is to not only seek the simple wants of life or what other people want you to do but always follow your true will. Unlike other religions, there are no guidelines for what will harm and what will not, leaving it entirely up to interpretation. Some Wiccan sects take the Wiccan Rede to mean not harm yourself. This sometimes also extends to animals and plants but will disregard other people. Overall, the interpretation of the Rede is up to the Wiccan. Still, it is commonly understood that it encourages people to take responsibility for their actions and not to harm another person or thing.

The Rule of Three

Occultists, Neopagans, and Wiccans follow the tenet of the Rule of Three, which states that the energy a person puts into the world will return to the person three times. The Rule of Three pertains to both positive and negative energies, which can help to deter Wiccans from practicing dark magick. Although some Wiccans call the Rule of Three karma, they are not the same concept. However, they both encourage a person to do good, and good will be done to them in return.

Some Wiccans do not take the Rule of Three literally. Instead, they believe energy will return to them as often as possible until they learn the lesson they need. The ideas of the three also relate to the Triple Goddess. Although not all Wiccans adhere to the Rule of Three, some believe it was created to mimic Christianity.

The Rede and Rule of Three are two fundamental Wiccan beliefs that different sects can variably interpret. By looking at these practices, it is evident that speeches and poems are often reinterpreted, with their resulting practices reflecting these shifts in understanding. In the next chapter, we will discuss the numerous holidays and their significance to Wicca.

5

Holidays and Festivals

Deities and magick are essential parts of the Wiccan belief and practice. As we know, the Triple Goddess and Horned God are beings integral to the Wiccan religion, and a part of their worship is through holidays and festivals. Like any religion, holidays and festivals are vital parts of their practice. Historically, religions had numerous festivals that served many different purposes. Looking at the ancient Greeks had festivals that were meant to appease Demeter so that people would have healthy crops and abundant harvests. They had gathered for Dionysus, and they would worship him through drinking, feasting, and having sex. There were festivals for the transition of children from childhood to adulthood. As with past religions, Wiccans have many festivals and holidays. Although nowadays, when we think about holidays, Christmas and Halloween are likely to come to our minds, the festivals and holidays which the Wiccans practice are not the same. In this chapter, we will explore many of them and what their purpose is.

Wheel of the Year

The Wheel of the Year is a symbol used to show the eight sabbats in which Wiccans participate throughout the year. A thousand years ago, Celts celebrated the festivals present on the Wheel of the Year that Wiccans use today. However, there is no proof of an ancient Wheel of the Year used during the ancient times, as some Wiccans try to claim. The names of the festivals the Celts celebrated differ from those of the Wiccans.

The passing of time and life is captured in the Wheel of the Year. It is a reminder that nothing is ever-lasting but also an affirmation of eternal return and rebirth. And although the seasons change and people die, everything comes around again. This goes along with the Wiccan belief in rebirth or reincarnation. Even if someone's physical body might die, their soul is reborn into a new body. Despite modernization changing ideas around time being linear, the Wheel of the Year and its celebrations allow them to connect with nature and accept their time as it is.

Greater or Eight Sabbats

Through the eight sabbats, Wiccans can honor their connection with nature. Represented by the Wheel of the Year, these seasonal celebrations provide an opportunity to reflect on our place in the world and come together in harmony. Although you might think, why are there eight celebrations when there are only four seasons? This is because they mark the beginning and middle of each season. Despite many Wiccans practicing in solitary rather than in a coven, the greater sabbats keep time for everyone to get together and connect with other Wiccans and nature. The cyclical nature of time represented in the eight sabbats allows Wiccans to reflect on what they have gained and lost in the past year. Reflecting on gratitude and looking toward the future, but also reflecting on the past, allows Wiccans to find balance and harmony in their lives.

Samhain (October 31)

Although each of the sabbats falls on a day or a couple of days to which the Wiccans hold significance, Samhain is one of the most important. For Wicca, Samhain marks the beginning of a new year, like the New Year's Day that most people celebrate on January 1st. The name Samhain means summer's end and is especially important because it occurs on the last day of the season of light and marks the beginning of the darkness. Yet, misconceptions persist that the season of darkness is inherently evil, particularly in light of Halloween. But this is incorrect; darkness and light to Wiccans are not symbols of good and evil but necessities. One cannot have light without regenerative darkness. Symbols of light and dark, the Horned God and the Triple Goddess, are neither good nor bad. Instead, they emphasize our interconnectedness with nature and remind us that there is a balance between two opposite forces.

Samhain was celebrated throughout history as ancient sites in Ireland, Wales, Scotland, and Britain all showed gathering sites for Samhain. While non-Wiccans do not typically observe Samhain, many of its older practices resemble today's Halloween traditions. Bonfires on Halloween and many practices of mischief night have been traced back to the practices of Samhain. As the bonfires were lit, sacrifices such as crops and animals were burned, which is a protective measure against evil spirits. And nowadays, people will burn bonfires to symbolize this meaning.

During this festival, Wiccans took a moment to reflect on the past year and honor those who had been lost and their ancestors. Wicca, along with many other cultures, believed that the veil between the lands of the living and dead was the thinnest on Samhain, which allowed the dead to traverse the land of the living easily. Although this might have been frightening for some, Wiccans believed it allowed ancestors and departed loved ones to communicate with the living. One custom for this was to make the favorite meal for those who had died. However, spirits being able to cross the veil also meant that those who felt as though they were wronged could seek compensation or retribution.

Meanwhile, traveling at night on Samhain was warned against as it was believed that non-human spirits, such as fairies and sprites, lived in the spirit world and could cross over into the human realm to seduce and abduct mortals that were not being careful. And to protect their identity, people use masks and costumes to ward off spiritual beings that seek to do them harm.

Yule, The Winter Solstice (December 20-25)

Yule is the sabbat celebrating the shortest day of the year, the Winter Solstice. This day is significant to the Wiccans as it represents the renewing nature of life's cycles because the length of the day only prolongs after this festivity. Pagans use Yule to celebrate the birth of a Sun God. And for Wiccans, this same date marks the reincarnation of the Horned God at the hands of the Triple Goddess. So, on Yule, Wiccans take special notice of the evergreen tree, decorating it in honor of the Sun or Horned God and leaving gifts for him. Among Wiccans, the evergreen stands for life's strength and ability to endure despite changing seasons.

Alongside the evergreen tree, a bonfire is lit to burn the Yule log. Once again, a bonfire is present during the season of darkness to resemble rebirth and new beginnings. Each year, a piece of the Yule log is saved for the next year, and as people sang around the fire, they would throw holly into it. The holly was meant to symbolize the challenges that they have been experiencing and how they will not weigh them down but help them to grow.

Now, let us discuss the two figures in Wicca: The Oak King and Holly King. The Yule celebration is to show the Oak King coming back into power over the Holly King. These two figures stand for light and darkness. As the days become shorter and there is less light, the Holly King rules, and the Oak king rules when the days are longer. The exchange of power between these two shows the continuity of life.

Imbolc (February 1-2)

Sitting halfway between the Winter Solstice and Spring Equinox, this festival is a time to celebrate purification and rebirth. Imbolc means in the belly, which signifies fertility, promise for the future, and hope. The Celtic goddess Brigid is often symbolized during this festival, as she was the goddess of fertility, poetry, medicine, sacred springs, and the forge. Some Wiccans will make dolls in the goddess' likeness by weaving cornstalk. Making these gifts in her honor was meant to represent continuity, luck, and fertility. February 2nd is relevant even to non-Wiccans, as in Western society, Groundhog Day occurs. Wiccans would celebrate Imbolc in the hope of an early spring.

Ostara, The Spring Equinox (March 20-23)

The promise of hope, birth, and fertility is met when Wiccans celebrate Ostara, also known as the Spring Equinox. In history, Ostara has been sacred to Pagans. Still, their celebrations were kept secret, and very little is known about how Pagans would celebrate Ostara before Jacob Grimm brought it to light. Eostre, the Germanic goddess of spring and fertility, inspired the holiday's name. Like Persephone, Eostre was said to rise from the earth on the equinox, bringing spring with her. Different myths say that she either sleeps during the months before or is pregnant and gives birth as she leaves the earth. The Triple Goddess is depicted as becoming impregnated by the Horned God around this time. This sabbat emphasizes renewal and rebirth, yet little is known about how Wiccans commemorate it. Evidence suggests that feasting, which may sometimes include a rabbit, was part of the festivities.

Beltane (April 30 - May 01)

Beltane is a festival that occurs in the middle of spring and celebrates fertility, light, and the coming of summer. Bel, the Celtic god, is believed to be the inspiration for the name as it comes from the phrase "Bel's Fire," which means bright fire. Bonfires are essential during this festival, as fire is associated with passion. During this festival, people are meant to indulge in their desires and set aside their inhibitions.

During ancient Pagan rituals, dancing around a tree and wrapping ribbons around a maypole were performed. A young woman would also be picked to become the May Queen, who was meant to stand in for the fertility goddess Flora.

This festival signifies the increase of light in the world as nature continues to awaken. However, this also means unseen awakening entities within the spirit realm. Although fairies were typically seen as being safe, they were also known to be mischief makers. The ritual of placing a rowan branch in the house's ceiling was performed by the head of the home, as well as a cleansing, which involved carrying a lit candle from the front door to the back door, to the corners of the house, and from the hearth to one side of the main rooms. The walking around symbolizes the creation of a net with eight points.

Litha, The Summer Solstice (June 20-22)

As the year's longest day draws near, it is marked by the celebration of the Summer Solstice or the Litha sabbat. This celebration makes the official transition of power from the Oak King to the Holly King. After this day, the days start to become shorter. Dancing, bonfires, feasting, honey cakes, and fresh fruits are traditional at this festival. However, this festival is celebrated as light triumphing over darkness, despite knowing that darkness would slowly overtake light again after that day.

At the Summer Solstice, individuals protect themselves from unseen dangers, like spirit entities. It is believed that these mystical forces began to stir during Beltane and are at their peak when summer arrives, causing harm to those who do not take preventive measures. To protect oneself from such external forces, rituals are conducted all day long at Litha Sabbat, and sun wheels made of stalks are crafted as a symbol of this celebration. If one was married on this day, protection rituals were especially performed on the couples to ensure their marriages were happy and healthy.

Lughnasadh (August 1)

This festival is named after the Celtic god of truth and order, Lugh. Known as a harvest festival, Lughnasadh focuses on the passing of summer and the coming of fall. The Horned God's death is seen as approaching, and he would return to Summerland and the underworld until the Triple Goddess brought him back. During this festival, fruits and vegetables would be harvested; the first offered to the gods and goddesses.

Harvest, fall, and death also link to the god Lugh and the myth of him and his foster mother, Tailtiu. She was one of the first Celtic gods, and her tale depicts her dutifully and selflessly slowing the land of Ireland to prepare it for its people; as a result, she died from exhaustion. To honor her, Lugh would hold an annual feast on her death, which became Lughnasadh.

Common activities during this sabbat include archery, horse racing, fencing, racing, boxing, and wrestling matches. These activities are funeral rituals to honor Tailtiu, but they also were used as a final celebration of summer.

Mabon, The Autumn Equinox (September 20-23)

Mabon, the celebration of the Autumn Equinox, completes the wheel of the world and is used as a time for reflection and giving thanks. Unlike many other sabbats, the name is a modern invention, first being named in the 1970s. It has been observed that nearly every ancient civilization had a figure that would descend into the underworld as a marking of autumn and winter approaching and then reemerge at the beginning of spring. Depending on the religion, a god or goddess would be seen as dying on this day and returning to the underworld. For Wiccans, this would be the Horned God. Other examples include Persephone from ancient Greece.

During the Mabon sabbat, Wiccans and Pagans will celebrate the second harvest and the coming of winter. Giving thanks for the crops they had been able to harvest that year was especially important during this sabbat. Celebrating the gifts, they could gather from the forest also comes with the acknowledgment that the soil was dying for the winter seasons.

Esbat

Aside from the greater or eight sabbats, there are other festivals and celebrations known as Esbats that Wiccans participate in. Every month, when the full moon rises, people meet and celebrate together in groups or by themselves for Esbats. These gatherings are an opportunity to take part in initiations and healing magick. The thirteen lunar months of the year are all marked by Esbats, making each full moon a special occasion.

Wiccans often observe Esbats during the full moon. Yet, specific covens or practitioners may also choose to celebrate them at new moons. Esbats are essential as covens or individuals will draw power from the moon, allowing others to feel empowered during these times. During new moon Esbats, rituals are performed for healing, personal growth, and initiation into new ventures. They are the most intimate among the celebrations, and outsiders are rarely invited.

Gods and goddesses are still honored during Esbats, although not as much as with sabbats. Traditionally, during an Esbat, a circle would be cast. But if a coven or singular person does not do this purifying, alternative purification methods, such as smudging, are performed in specific areas. Doing this marks the place as sacred. Bowls of water and moon candles are essential to the rituals performed during an Esbat. More on Wiccan rituals will be explored later in the book.

As you have learned, there are numerous festivals, holidays, and rituals that Wiccans partake in throughout the year, and this does not include any personal ones that a coven or person might practice, including those around birth, marriage, and death, which will be discussed in the next chapter.

6

Birth, Marriage, and Death

Each religion and person have a way of celebrating or grieving. And within Wicca, there might be different ways that different types of Wiccans perform rituals. Besides celebrating Sabbats and Esbats, there are numerous other rituals; Wiccans participate, either in a coven or individually, including birth, marriage, separation, death, and the afterlife. In this chapter, we will look at how Wiccans perform rituals of wiccaning, handfasting, hand parting, crossing the bridge, and afterlife and reincarnation.

Birth Rite (Wiccaning)

If you are a part of the Pagan community and have a child, you will likely hear whether you will have a wiccaning ceremony for your child. You can also be new to the Pagan community and hear whether you will have a wiccaning ceremony for yourself. It is important to remember that not all Pagans are Wiccans; you can be part of the Pagan community but not be a Wicca. The wiccaning ceremony welcomes an infant, child, or new person into the Pagan or Wiccan community. It is often compared to baptism for Christians.

Pagans who do not identify as Wiccan go through their welcoming ceremony called saining. You do not need to go through a wiccaning to be a Wiccan, nor do you need to perform this ceremony for your children. It is entirely up to you as a person or parent whether you want to have a wiccaning.

Saining is very similar to wiccaning, and during this, charms will be made for the child, and rituals to perform to ensure they remain safe and healthy throughout their lives. In ancient wiccaning and saining practices, there are writings of children being passed through a hole carved from stone, and the act was meant as a protective measure from fairies and other creatures in the spirit world. Protection from fairies was critical because Pagans believed that fairies would come to the mortal realm and kidnap babies, leaving a changeling in its place. A wiccaning or saining ceremony emphasizes the protection of children. Presenting a person or child to the gods and goddesses is traditional for a wiccaning ceremony.

It is important to remember that partaking in a wiccaning ceremony for yourself or your child does not mean you are locked into anything. A wiccaning is just a matter of welcoming you or someone else into a spiritual community where you will hopefully be able to grow and flourish.

Handfasting (Marriage)

Handfasting is a marriage ceremony that has existed for thousands of years and is present in numerous cultures; however, it is believed to have Celtic origins. Its origins are heavily tied to nature and spirituality and where the phrase "tying the knot" comes from when discussing marriage.

The history of handfasting predates Christianity, and since many people could not afford to buy gold rings for their spouses, a handfasting ceremony was a much more affordable option. Despite the ritual being nothing more than a ribbon, an old fabric, or a cord tied to the hands of two people as they exchange vows, it still felt deeply spiritual. Typically, the couple would keep their hands tied together until midnight. If they overcome their hardships while connected, their union will succeed. Yet, nowadays, the couple would typically only stay tied together for the ceremony.

The rope and fabric used in a handfasting ceremony carry different meanings. But it will be up to the couple to decide which symbols to impart. When selecting the colors, factors are considered, such as:

- past, present, and future
- dreams, adventures, and hopes
- promises you are making to one another
- personality
- special individuals in your life

Wiccans are the only community to practice handfasting. But if you are part of a coven, the coven leader will typically perform the handfasting ceremony. Several parts go into this ceremony, and they usually go in the following order:

- music and processional
- welcoming the guests and statement of intention
- first reading
- second reading
- presentation of cords or ribbons for handfasting
- ritual in which couples' hands are bound
- vow exchange
- declaration of marriage
- closing statement
- recessional and music

How your handfasting ceremony goes might differ depending on whether you are part of a coven, if you are also performing other rituals, or wish to include anything else in the ceremony. Alongside the ceremony, the couple and guests might partake in a tradition known as jumping a besom broom, which signifies the building of a home and hearth together.

For Wiccans, in particular, there are two stages of marriage. The first is betrothal, which lasts a year. At this time, the couple is given a chalice, and after the year, the couple performs the handfasting ritual. The chalice is also shattered during this ritual, and the couple is given the pieces.

Handparting (Separation)

Not everyone is meant to be married, and Wiccans recognize this; thus, they have hand parting rituals. Handparting is the rite that formally ends a handfasting, cutting the symbolic and spiritual ties established during the ceremony. This ritual also emphasizes that, although there is no longer emotional love between the couple, there is still a friendship. Wicca does not punish divorce as their marriage vows are as long as love shall last. There being no punishment or discrimination of divorce makes it much easier for a couple to separate, making their relationship outside of marriage much healthier.

If a couple is legally married, they will still need to undergo a civil divorce, and the handparting ceremony can occur any time before or after this happens. For Wiccans, handfasting can equate to marriage, but to be legally married, one would need to have a civil marriage and, thus, a divorce. If a couple does not have a civil union, the handparting ceremony equates to divorce.

Who attends this ceremony is wholly on a case-to-case basis. Some couples will want only a priest or priestess present, while others will wish to have parents, loved ones, and children if the situation is amicable.

The handparting ceremony will occur at an altar that can be set up in someone's home or the officiant's office. It will be covered in cobalt blue, black for wisdom, red for healing, and other cloth that might be meaningful to the couple. The shards of the chalice and the cords from their handfasting should be present during the ritual. Gods and deities are called on to oversee the ritual, and the couple will discuss the lessons they learned from the marriage. The goal of this ceremony is for the peaceful separation of the parties so that they may respect their former partner and the relationship they had.

Crossing the Bridge (Death)

As you can tell throughout this chapter, Wiccans have numerous rituals for different aspects of life, and one of the final ones is the crossing the bridge ritual performed at a Wiccan's death. Other Wiccan groups will perform this ceremony differently, but they all honor the death of a Wiccan with a crossing the bridge ritual. Some common rituals include a spiral dance representing the cycle of life or a reenactment of a god or goddess descending into the underworld. Storytelling, feasting, and drinking are also common funeral rites of Wiccans. The stories would typically reflect the life of the person who has passed on. Emphasis on life and death is essential during this ritual as it leads to the next aspect of Wiccan beliefs: the afterlife and reincarnation.

Afterlife and Reincarnation

As we learned in an earlier chapter, the Horned God is the ruler of the underworld, and Summerland is the realm where spirits wait to be reincarnated. Concepts of the afterlife and reincarnation are not new, as each culture and religion have its own. Depending on the culture, the aspect of a reborn human will differ, whether mind, soul, or consciousness. Although the afterlife and reincarnation are present within the Wiccan practices, not all Wiccans believe in them. Wiccan traditions are meant to make the most out of your life rather than dwelling on what will happen afterward. Depending on the Wiccan, some believe that humans can only be reincarnated into new human bodies, while others acknowledge that you could be reincarnated into an animal. When spirits were within Summerland, a medium could contact them.

Feri Wicca is one type of Wicca that has ideas about the soul and what happens afterward. It adopted the Hawaiian notion, which states human beings have three souls. This can connect back to the ideas of three with the Rule of Three and the Triple Goddess.

We have discussed numerous Wiccan beliefs, including deities, the elements, ethics, holidays and festivals, and numerous rituals that occur throughout a person's life. We have completed Pillar 2, and it is time to discuss Pillar 3, which is all about Wiccan practices, starting with the numerous ways you can practice Wicca.

Pillar 3
Practice

Many of us are drawn to Wicca for the freedom it offers. We each have our journey, and sometimes we must figure out which path to take. That is why Pillar 3, covering the practices of Wicca, is so essential; it focuses on what kind of practice you could pursue. Thus, this section will discuss Chapter 7, about choosing your practice, and Chapter 8, about getting initiated.

In Chapter 7, we explore the different types of practices within Wicca. You can choose from coven-based, solitary, hereditary, eclectic, hedge, secular, cosmic, green, kitchen, hearth, gray, or augury practices. Whichever one calls out to you will best fit your spiritual path.

Then, in Chapter 8, we will look at getting initiated into a particular tradition through coven initiation. There are two rites; the rite of dedication and the rite of passage. Through these rites comes transformation and an initiation into a new way of being in the world that may bring greater understanding and connection to yourself and deeper ties with others who are also on that path.

7

Choose your Practice

Depending on the type of religion you practice, there can be many different branches of that religion from which you can choose to practice. As we have learned, Wicca was formed by Gardner but did not force all Wiccans to practice the same way he did. Within Wicca, there are numerous ways you can practice because the primary goal of Wicca is connecting with yourself and nature; however, you choose to do so. As Wicca reached different parts of western culture, it was introduced to many people who adapted it to best suit them. This chapter will discuss some of the most common ways that Wicca is practiced.

Coven Based

When Wicca was founded, the primary way that it was practiced was through covens. Gardner formed one of the first covens at the beginning of Wicca, and as it exploded, it was the primary way witches practiced Wicca. A coven is a group of witches that gather to perform rituals and rites. For the sabbats, esbats, and rituals discussed in the previous section of this book, covens would gather for those. The number of witches within a coven would vary, and witches did not need to be related to form a coven. Three or more is considered a coven. The strength of a coven was not determined by the number of witches that were a part of it.

Instead, it was about their connection, nature, and power. Three powerful witches could be stronger than a coven of 10.

Solitary

As Wicca is not as popular as it used to be, it can be hard to find a coven, so many Wiccans decide to practice solitarily. A Wiccan might want to work alone as well. Not having a coven can give a witch some freedom because instead of following the coven's practices, you can combine different practices to do the best for you and allow yourself to make the deep connections you want.

Hereditary

Not all witches are born as such. Many Wiccans, especially when it was just created, were likely a part of another religion and decided to practice Wicca because they agreed with its core values and practices more. Hereditary witches are those that inherit their magick from their families. Many people born into Wiccan families likely identify in some regard as hereditary witches. These witches probably do not have rituals and practices solely based on their status as hereditary but are part of another type of Wicca.

Eclectic

Eclectic witches identify as Wiccan, but their practices and beliefs are not strictly Pagan. Instead, they adopt aspects of other religions and philosophies into their practices. Whether in a coven or not, the ideologies and religions you embrace will vary. There are no concrete rules to eclectic Wicca, which is why many Wiccans choose this type of practice.

Secular

Unlike other witches who rely on religion and spirituality to tap into their magical abilities, secular witches do not bind their power to any faith or mysticism. This means that they are free to practice their craft without the constraints of adhering to Wiccans' particular set of beliefs. Likewise, these witches are often distanced from the Wiccan tradition or any other faith-based practice and define themselves independently.

Cosmic

Cosmic witches focus on the stars, astronomy, and astrology as integral parts of their practice. The moon is a fundamental part of their rituals in all its phases, as it is with other Wicca forms. These aspects of cosmic witchcraft, which are present in many Wiccan rituals, add to the power of their practice. Usually, these witches use incantations and moon cycles for protection against celestial happenings. They have an affinity for star signs and birth charts in their craft. Likewise, they change energies using their extensive knowledge of the star signs and help people better understand themselves and the cosmos' influence on them.

Green

Green witches are those that specialize in healing, nature, and nurturing. Their power, rituals, and tools all come from the earth. Plant, flowers, and herbal preparations are commonly made by these witches and are a primary source of ingredients for different spells. These witches hold nature in the utmost regard and respect it above all else. Plus, they play a large part in sabbats around harvesting, healing, and fertility.

Hedge

Hedge witches share much in common with green witches, but while the latter dedicate their magick to nature, hedge witches can practice various forms of magick. Also, they often practice alone, and like eclectic witches, they do not limit themselves to one belief system. Instead, they can incorporate numerous spiritual and religious approaches in their work. Likewise, these witches keep everything basic and straightforward, as they often do not have the support of other coven members. They also focus their abilities on herbal remedies, the elements, and nature. The freedom that hedge witches have makes it viable for someone who is drawn to nature but does not want to be a part of a coven like most green witches are.

Kitchen

As the name suggests, kitchen witches focus their energy on the kitchen. They mix magick into their cooking and baking, utilizing herbs for their metaphysical properties. Every ingredient has been carefully chosen to ensure the best outcome for each dish, not just for flavor but also to unlock the potential of its magical qualities. When there are celebrations and festivals, kitchen witches prepare meals to share with the coven and external community. Depending on the purpose of the gathering, they will make different dishes.

Hearth

Hearth witches are similar to the kitchen and green witches but are centered around the home. These witches concentrate their abilities on rituals and objects around the house, including ritual cleansing, herbalism, and candle magick. They also have a vast knowledge of protection spells as they take it into their hands to protect the house.

Gray

White and dark magick is used through Wicca, with different types of witches leaning one side over the other. Yet, gray witches like to straddle the line between the two as they use whichever is best for the situation they find themselves in. Curses and hexes are typically considered dark magick, and while most witches will not use them, gray witches will if they think it is necessary. Although these witches use both forms of magick, they are not evil. Instead, they use dark magick to redirect bad energy and seek justice. They use their magick to call on unseen forces to help them correct unfair circumstances and injustices.

Augury

Augury witches can use their power to decipher omens, typically from the behaviors of birds, animals, and the weather. These witches are generally able to use divination as well. They might also call themselves prophets. Besides that, they could use the movement of birds, animals, or the weather to determine auspices, of which there are five different kinds:

- **Ex caelo = from the sky:** does not involve birds but looks toward thunder and lightning for the omens of the gods.
- **Ex avibus = from birds:** not all birds or animals were symbols of gods communicated. There were traditionally two ways augury witches could interpret, through song and their movement while flying. Common birds used for these practices included ravens, owls, hens, and crows.
- **Ex tripudiis = from birds feeding:** chickens were generally used for this practice. Augury witches would throw food at chickens; depending on how they reacted, it would be a good or bad omen.

- **Ex quadrupedibus = from quadrupeds:** omens were taken from animals that walked on four legs, such as a dog, fox, wolf, or horse.
- **Ex diris = from portents:** these are the least likely to be used as they are not from weather or animals but are essentially any action that seems to be abnormal.

These are just a few of the many Wiccan practices you can choose from. You can even select a few different ones and decide which rituals, forms, and practices you want. No matter where you are drawn, there are so many other Wiccan practices that you can adopt. The next part of Pillar 3, after you have chosen your practice, is getting initiated into Wicca. You might be surprised to learn that there are multiple ways to begin.

8

Get Initiated

Now that you know the history of Wicca and its foundations and have chosen which Wiccan practice you would like to focus on, it is time to get initiated into Wicca. Initiation into Wicca is different from the wiccaning we talked about earlier. Being welcomed into the spiritual side of Wicca through a wiccaning does not imply any commitment to practicing Wicca. Yet, one way to become initiated is by performing a ritual where you are devoted to it. But this does not mean someone is forced to stay within Wicca; you can leave Wicca and a coven whenever you desire. There are two ways that you can become initiated into Wicca: coven initiation or self-dedication.

Coven Initiation

During the start of Wicca, taking part in a coven initiation was how the majority became Wiccan. This is because very few people would know about Wiccan practices without being part of the community unless they were looking for it. Unlike larger and more widespread religions, information about Wicca was not easily accessible like it is today, making coven initiation the go-to. Coven initiations do not occur as much today as many Wiccans practice solitarily rather than as part of a coven. This is because the number of Wiccan covens has significantly decreased since its beginning. However, there are still a few covens, however small they may be. To take part in a coven initiation, there are two rites in which you have to partake. The first is the rite of dedication, and the second is the rite of passage. It is important to note that although all covens have these two rites, there can be different ways of performing them. And each coven might have various rites or rituals that need to be completed by initiated members to become fully integrated into the coven.

Rite of Dedication

The rite of dedication is used to signify when someone wants to join a coven. After Wiccans performed this dedication, they start to train with the coven. Depending on the coven, how long the training period goes on will differ. The meaning of this dedication to the person and the coven will vary based on the circumstances. Some covens might take it very seriously, while others might not as much. The training after the proper ritual is performed can also be considered part of the rite as initiates learn the rules and skills of the coven. During the dedication, a witch is learning to embody all the coven stands for.

Going through a rite of dedication can change someone's curiosity about Wicca and its beliefs to a commitment to learning the practices and developing their own identity. Under the lunar light, this is an opportunity for initiates to connect with nature and have the direct attention of the gods while dedicating themselves to Wiccan teachings.

Rite of Passage

After someone has gone through the rite of dedication, they can go through their rite of passage. The rite of passage into a coven usually occurs a year and a day after their rite of dedication. Typically, it is a ceremonial event in which the person or people performing it must execute different tasks or rituals to complete the rite. Across the ages and in many other societies, rites of passage have been observed. The extent of this ceremony and everything that goes into it will differ depending on your coven. For such, the rite of passage's cultural, social, and psychological significance may vary. Going through this process allows a person to gain acceptance into society. As for Wiccans, this means that the witch or witches performing the ceremony will be initiated into the coven upon completion.

Depending on whether you are born into Wicca or find it later in life, your rite of passage will be different. For those born Wiccan, their rites of passage are likely connected to bodily milestones like puberty or entering adulthood. However, when you find Wicca later in life, your rite might be based on how long you have been practicing. The type of rite of passage you perform will differ from coven to coven. For any rite of passage, the goal is to purify the person and prepare them to start the next part of their life as a Wiccan. The purification that is performed allows individuals to communicate with the supernatural and connect with nature. For someone not born into Wicca, the cleansing of this rite can symbolize the shedding of your past life and the beginning of your new one as a Wiccan.

Social transformations, like coming of age or being inducted into a coven, are also part of the rite of passage. Here is a breakdown of the different rites of passage you might experience.

Life Cycle Ceremonies

Each coven will have different life cycle ceremonies. These rites of passage are linked to biological milestones in a person's life, including birth, childhood, and transitioning into adulthood. Depending on the coven you are in and their practice, you could go through numerous life cycle ceremonies, and there could be different rites for different sexes. Depending on the type of magick they use and their practices, the events and what is performed can differ significantly.

Social Transformation Ceremonies

Social transformation also encompasses the life cycle ceremonies as people transition from one stage of their life to another. These transitions also cause their social status and roles to change. Ceremonies outside those connected to life cycles do not have a connection to biological milestones but occur as someone's social role transforms. An example of a social transformation as a rite of passage would be someone being initiated into the coven as a new Wiccan, or it could be when someone's role in the coven is changed, such as a new coven leader being put into power.

Religious Transformation Ceremonies

Sacrifices and offerings are very common during these ceremonies to symbolize everything a person is giving up and what they are willing to give. Someone who is not a Wiccan, being initiated into a coven, would experience a religious transformation during their rite of passage.

Self-Dedication

Wicca today is very different from what it was even 20 years ago. Covens were much more prominent then and accessible to people looking to be initiated into Wicca. However, finding covens is much more challenging nowadays, especially ones publicly looking for more initiates. Meanwhile, self-dedication became much more recognized, allowing you to practice the way you want and not need to follow the rules of a coven. As we discussed, covens would perform the rites and rituals for a proper initiation, but you must execute them alone during self-dedication. You cannot initiate yourself into Wicca because this would mean there would be other witches performing the ceremony; this is why it is called a dedication rather than an initiation.

Although it is not necessary for you to perform a self-dedication ceremony, doing so is an excellent way of solidifying your relationship with the gods, goddesses, nature, and the Divine. When and how you choose to dedicate yourself to Wicca will depend on you. Some people like to study for one year and a day and then devote themselves; others will choose specific times in the year or the month to do so. It is entirely up to you how you choose to dedicate yourself to Wicca. Yet, even if you can decide when and how to commit yourself, it is essential to take time because it is a significant part of your spiritual journey. Here is an example of a simple self-dedication ritual that you can change to fit your needs better.

The Wiccan practice of self-dedication is traditionally performed in a state of nudity. For instance, being naked during the ritual represents a sincere vulnerability and openness to the divine forces and the self. Likewise, it is believed to remove any barriers that may hinder the practitioner's connection with their inner essence, as well as with the natural world and the divine energies. However, if being naked is impossible, alternative conditions are provided for the ritual. These conditions include ensuring that the area is free of distractions, private, and quiet. Both options aim to create an environment conducive to focused and uninterrupted ritual practice. To complete this ritual, you will need blessing oil, salt, and a white candle. Begin by grounding yourself through meditation. Allow your mind to relax, and do not focus on anything mundane. Once settled, pour salt onto the ground and stand in it. Have the white candle close enough to feel its heat when you light it. Look into the flame of the candle and think about your motivations as you follow this script to complete your self-dedication:

Stand by the altar and say: *"I am a child of the gods, and I ask them to bless me."*

Dip your finger into the blessing oil, and with your eyes closed, anoint your forehead. Some people trace a pentagram on the skin with the oil. Say: "May my mind be blessed so I can accept the wisdom of the gods." Anoint the eyelids (be careful here!) and say: *"May my eyes be blessed, so I can see my way clearly upon this path."*

Anoint the tip of your nose with the oil, and say: *"May my nose be blessed, so I can breathe in the essence of all that is Divine."*

Anoint your lips, and say: *"May my lips be blessed, so I may always speak with honor and respect."*

Anoint your chest, and say: *"May my heart be blessed, so I may love and be loved."*

Anoint the tops of your hands, and say: *"May my hands be blessed so that I may use them to heal and help others."*

Anoint your genital area, and say: *"May my womb be blessed so that I may honor the creation of life."* (If you are male, make the appropriate changes here.)

Anoint the soles of your feet, and say: *"May my feet be blessed so that I may walk side by side with the Divine."*

If you have specific deities you follow, pledge your loyalty to them now. Otherwise, you can use *"God and Goddess"* or *"Mother and Father."* Say: *'Tonight, I pledge my dedica-*

> *tion to the God and Goddess. I will walk with them beside me and ask them to guide me on this journey. I pledge to honor them and ask that they allow me to grow closer to them. As I will, so it shall be"* (Wigington, 2018c).

This is just one way you can perform the self-dedication ritual. Because it is you and you alone performing it, you can change it however you want. What matters is that you are fully allowing yourself to become dedicated to Wicca and that this ceremony best suits your desires for your experience as a Wiccan. Do not let others dictate how you dedicate yourself to Wicca. The self-dedication ritual I gave you above is simple. If you want something more extravagant, make it so; if you are going to keep it as simple as possible, do it. You can include other rituals in this as well.

Whether a coven initiates you or you go down the path of self-dedication, you are now a full member of Wicca. Now that you have chosen your practice and are a full member, it is time to dive into Pillar 4 and discuss the various forms of magick.

Pillar 4
Magick

In pillar 4, we will explore Wiccan's magick, an ancient, mysterious, and powerful practice with many layers. Also, we will delve into three different chapters about natural magick, ceremonial magick, and celestial magick, each of which has unique aspects to explore.

Starting with natural forces in chapter 9, we will learn how to perform rituals and spells using plants, herbs, animals, crystals, and more. Then we will soon uncover the core elements of ceremonial magick in chapter 10 and techniques for summoning spirits. And finally, in chapter 11, celestial magick will be discussed on how it relates to the divine.

As we explore pillar 4, more of its components will be unveiled. Now, let us dive deeper into the mystery that awaits us in the upcoming chapters.

9

Natural Magick

There are three different kinds of magick that a Wiccan can use. The first kind that we are going to talk about is natural magick. As the name sounds, this magick draws on the natural world. Wiccans believe there are two worlds, the natural and the spirit, and to draw on these worlds requires different magick. Natural magick is used for the human world and uses different plants, herbs, animals, crystals, and other natural forces to perform various rituals, potions, and spells.

Although the word magick is attached to the name, much of natural magick is drawn from natural sciences, such as alchemy, astronomy, astrology, chemistry, and botany. And even if Wicca is modern in its invention, natural magick has been around since the Renaissance. When using natural magick, many different flowers, herbs, fruits, and crystals are used, which people call upon for their magick properties. Depending on the purpose of your magick, the substances you use will change. Throughout this chapter, we will learn about natural magick materials, practices, and rituals.

The Elements and Plants

We learned earlier in this book the importance of elements for Wiccans, and now we have come back full circle. The elements are a central part of natural magick, and in the next chapter, they will also play a large role in ceremonial magick and summoning spirits. You might wonder why the elements and plants are together in one category. You might assume that plants would naturally fall under the category of earth. Still, following the writings of Agrippa in the 17th century, different parts of the plant are associated with other elements: the roots to earth, the leaves to water, the flowers to air, and the seeds to fire (Ball, 283). The thickness of the roots and being buried in the earth connects them to the element of the earth. Then, the leaves are connected to water because they contain juices. Meanwhile, flowers are connected to the air because of their subtlety. And the seeds are connected to fire, an element associated with passion and reproduction because this is how the flowers spread and grow.

Depending on the area that a Wicca lived, their access to different plants would be varied, but here are some of the most commonly used plants and their magickal properties.

Acacia

Acacia is also known as gum Arabic or Arabic gum and is associated with money, platonic love, spiritual and psychic enhancement, and protection. It can be used in many different ways, including incense. Augury witches, or those specializing in divination, used acacia to promote a meditative state, allowing them to interpret omens and messages more clearly. Protective elements of this herb make it helpful in storing ritual tools to ensure they are not corrupted or stolen by someone. This herb will also be prepared with oil to anoint censers and candles to help boost their spiritual and psychic abilities and protect them.

Bergamot

Bergamot is an herb that is traditionally used for burning during rituals to promote success. Bergamot was burned as it was believed to strengthen its power, versus if it was crushed and used in a potion. The burning aspect of this ritual and its strength can be related to modern-day aromatherapy, as burning would release the scent of bergamot, enhancing its ability. This herb is associated with money, prosperity, improving memory, promoting a better night's sleep, stopping inference, and protecting one from illness and evil. One can burn a bit of bergamot near their bedside for sleep benefits. Getting a better night's sleep is shown to improve memory as well. If you do not have access to fresh bergamot, using essential oil can give you some of the benefits it is associated with.

Berries

A multiple of berries are used in natural magick during rituals, but their primary use did not lie in their magickal abilities. Instead, it was left as an offering for gods, goddesses, and spirits. Strawberries are commonly used because of their bright coloring. How ripe and bright a berry determined the wealth of the crop, and the best-looking ones were made as an offering. Appeasing the gods, goddesses, and spirits with fruit helped ensure continued protection and fertility of the land.

Bluebells

Bluebells were used for many reasons, but one of the most common was to determine how psychically polluted the world was becoming. It was believed that bluebells would disappear as the world became more polluted. However, bluebells were known to be connected to witches, and people would no longer plant them, especially during witch hunts. Traditionally, it is said that witches could hear bluebells ringing if they had a visitor, which is why they would be planted near the door.

Deadly Nightshade

Poisonous plants are also used in natural magick, and deadly nightshade is one of the most commonly used. During ancient times, it was used as a preparation for anesthetics and poisons. For witchcraft, deadly nightshade is soaked in fat from an animal to create a cream that was said to promote astral projection. Astral projections could be used to help decipher messages from the gods. Nowadays, this type of potion is not used because the astral projections witches claimed to have are now known to be hallucinations caused by the deadly nightshade.

Eyebright

Another herb that is connected to divination and clairvoyance is eyebright. This plant was used to create an eyewash that would help to develop a witch's ability to perform telepathy. To make this eyewash, you will need about two handfuls of eyebrights, a heatproof bowl, a bottle, and boiling water. Follow these steps to create your eyewash:

1. Add herbs and water into the bowl.
2. Stir the mixture until the herbs are coated and allow to infuse for a minimum of 10 minutes. The longer you let it infuse, the more powerful the mixture will be.
3. If you choose to, this is the time to invoke a spirit or deity.
4. Once the water has cooled, pour it into a bottle.

To use, rinse your eyes with the wash and perform the desired rituals.

Ginger

Ginger root is typically dried and ground into a powder to be used in spells and rituals. The herb is aromatic and used to spice rituals and spells and get results quicker. It was believed that putting ginger in food offered to the gods would make effects happen faster and stronger.

Lady's Mantel

Alchemy is one of the natural sciences used in natural magick, and lady's mantel was one of the herbs used in alchemy. It was believed that glassy beads of liquid that accumulated on the leaves of this herb overnight were used to create the philosopher's stone because the fluid was infused with the herb's magickal properties at a concentrated level. Likewise, the stone was believed to have healing properties that could prolong life, cure disease, and turn metals into gold. Witches using natural magick could try to remake the philosopher's stone.

Mugwort

Dream pillows and incense meant for divination typically had mugwort in them, the herb believed to aid in prophecy. However, its potency and power meant that it was used with caution, so it was only used as an infusion sparingly.

Vervain

Vervain also went by enchanter's herb and was used primarily to protect against negative energy and evil spells and purify sacred places and items, including homes, temples, altars, and tools. This herb dates back to ancient times, with the Egyptians, Greeks, and Romans using it for its magickal properties.

Crystals and Stones

Like plants, not all crystals and stones are linked to the earth. And so various types of crystals and stones correspond with different elements, making it essential to know which crystal is associated with which element when planning spells or rituals. Looking at each element, here are the crystals associated with them:

- **Air:** Clear stones and crystals. Yellow-tinged crystals are found to be okay, but they should be as clear as possible. Quartz is very commonly used. Imperfections in the crystal do not matter. As it is associated with air, imperfections or flaws are often compared to clouds in the sky.
- **Fire:** Stones and crystals associated with fire typically range in colors like orange, red, and black. Those crystals linked with volcanoes signify the fire that originated from within the earth.
- **Water:** Blue-green and blue stones and crystals are to be used for water. Pebbles found near water that are white or gray can also be used. These stones and crystals do not need to be polished. Besides that, pieces of salt or sand-blasted glass can also be used.
- **Earth:** Green and brown crystals and stones are recommended. As all stones and crystals are products of the earth, you want to make sure you distinguish them as being for the earth.
- **Spirit:** Purple stones and crystals, such as amethyst, are often used to represent the fifth element. Amethyst is considered one of the best crystals because it's a transmitter and receiver of spiritual and psychic energy.

To use stones and crystals for natural magick, there are a few things you need to understand and know about them. Stones and crystals have a way of speaking to witches to draw their attention. Yet, you might be drawn to them because of their shape or appearance. But as a Wiccan, you must trust your intuition and listen to which stones and crystals are calling you. When picking a suitable stone or crystal, ensure that you can comfortably hold it and fit it into your pocket. Once you have found the perfect stones or crystals for your needs, you must learn their story and how to use them properly. Different stones and crystals have other uses; it is up to you to determine those.

First, you must consider how the stone or crystal came to be in your possession. Ask yourself what it might have been before you picked it up. Was it larger and weathered over time, or was it broken off a larger piece? What has the stone or crystal experienced to get to you? When thinking about these questions, use your imagination first. But you will soon find that as your relationship with the stone and crystal grows, it will start giving you information and telling you its story. Your crystal's journey can be used to help you find the way through your own life.

After discovering its story, it is time to consider how and why you connected with it. Crystals and stones are packed with energy. They were once a gaseous material compacted into shape by energetic forces. The forces and energy within the crystals and stones can send out vibrations that can call to you, forming a connection.

Stones and crystals can have many benefits for the users, which you need to be aware of. The best way to ensure your crystals and stones are perfect for the natural magick you are trying to use is to understand the benefits you can get from them. Here are some of the benefits your stones and crystals can give you:

- **Can be used as an energizer:** Establishing a relationship with a crystal or stone can act as a mental and physical stimulant. When feeling exhausted, down, or disconnected, rubbing the stone can bring back feelings of stability and renew any lost connections, allowing you to tap into its energies again.

- **Can help you ground yourself:** Your stone or crystal can be used as a foundation for your journey. It can help ground you and support you in pursuing your goals effectively. Likewise, they can always remind you that we are all from the same earth, which is something to be grateful about.
- **Connect you to eternal wisdom:** We do not always recognize how much time and unseen forces go into the formation of stones and crystals. But for a crystal or stone to reach you, it can take some time, like how we exist on earth because of numerous decisions and hidden powers coming together.
- **Protection from harm:** Challenges coming in harm's way occur in everyone's lives, and your stone and crystal can help you work through your challenges. Your crystal and stone can help to remind you that you have the strength to weather the storms you are facing and stand tall against adversity. Many crystals and stones are believed to be able to protect against evil as well.
- **Can be used as a meditative aid:** Your stone or crystal can help you reach a peaceful state of mind, aiding your meditation.
- **A reminder that you are a part of a larger whole:** Your crystal or stone is one minuscule part of a larger whole. No matter where your crystal or stone originated, it was once a part of a larger whole, the same way you are. You are one part of your coven or one part of your family. You are one part of the world in itself. You can also make your stone or crystal a repository for your desires and dreams, which you can use to reflect on what you want from life.

Here are some common crystals and their known properties:

- **Clear quartz** helps to balance energy and amplify it, as well as aid in concentration and memory.
- **Rose quartz** helps enhance connections, restore trust and harmony in relationships, provide calm and comfort, and encourage respect, love, faith, and self-worth.
- **Obsidian** helps to remove emotional blockages, helps with finding one's true self, and promotes compassion, strength, and clarity.
- **Jasper** empowers the spirit, protects against negativity, promotes quick thinking, confidence, and courage, and supports you through times of stress.
- **Citrine** encourages warmth, optimism, motivation, and clarity, encourages creativity, supports concentration, and helps you release negative emotions.
- **Amethyst** helps rid of negative thoughts, promotes healthy choices and willpower, aids sleep, and allows for serenity, spiritual wisdom, and humility.
- **Turquoise** helps balance emotions and supports spiritual groundedness and good luck.
- **Bloodstone** encourages the circulation of energy and ideas, promotes creativity, idealism, and selflessness, and reduces aggressiveness, impatience, and irritability.
- **Ruby** restores energy levels and vitality, supports intellectual pursuit, brings recognition of truth and self-awareness, and promotes sensuality and sexuality.

Preparing a Circle with Stones and Crystals

Later in the book, we will discuss how to prepare magick circles, but one of the many ways is to use stones and crystals. You will want to arrange the different crystals and the elements they represent in the right spiritual direction. Here are some examples of crystals you can use for your magick circles:

- **North:** emerald, olivine, salt, moss agate, and black tourmaline
- **East:** imperial topaz, pumice, citrine, and mica
- **South:** obsidian, ruby, garnet, lava, amber, and rhodochrosite
- **West:** chalcedony, lapis lazuli, jade, sugilite, aquamarine, and moonstone

Depending on the circle size, you will put 7, 9, 21, or 40 stones in the circle, starting and ending at the beginning of the northern side. The number is significant because they serve to enhance your power. Some will also use ribbons or cords for their circle, which the stones can be placed on the inside or outside. The purpose of the ritual will also play a part in the direction of your crystals or stones. For rituals that send your power outwards, the points of your stones and crystals will face outwards, and protective ones will have the points inwards.

Natural magick can be potent, but it can also be nurturing and allow you to connect with yourself and nature on a level you did not think was possible. Many people are unaware of how much power the earth has because they do not open themselves to it. In the next chapter, we will discuss the second type of magick that someone can practice: ceremonial magick.

10
Ceremonial Magick

When someone says they practice ceremonial magick, this could mean they are performing a variety of different magicks because it is an encompassing term that can refer to various rituals and techniques. Traditionally, this magick requires the witch to use accessories that aid their magick. And like natural magick, it has been used for centuries and is believed to be originated during the Renaissance period. But they still have differences, as ceremonial magick requires both natural and external elements. Ceremonial magick is also used to summon gods and spirits. Throughout this chapter, we will discuss the numerous components of ceremonial magick, techniques, and the spirits that might be summoned.

Components of Ceremonial Magick

The components used in natural magick are all nature-based, including the elements, plants, crystals, and stones. Yet, for ceremonial magick, you need to use artificial ingredients, which help to enhance the user's magickal ability. Users will use four pieces: grimoires, magickal formulae, magickal weapons, and vibration of god names.

Grimoires are magick textbooks that every witch using ceremonial magick will carry. These grimoires contain spells, rituals, and instructions on creating amulets and talismans, summoning gods and spirits, and performing spells appropriately. Depending on the witches and covens, grimoires are believed to be imbued with magickal abilities. But covens and solitary witches use grimoires differently. Often, a single grimoire is kept by the leader of a coven. Or, by chance, they may present one to a witch when they come of age. Meanwhile, solitary witches who have access to a grimoire can choose what they do with it.

Magickal formulae, or 'words of power,' are individual words believed to possess supernatural or invocation abilities. These words encapsulate the levels of understanding and principles necessary to achieve a specific spell or ritual. Although they do not often fit into the context of sentences, they are meant to communicate abstract ideas. And while a single word or sentence may have little meaning, breaking it down into individual parts can give it much greater significance. Likewise, groupings of letters signify deeper sequences with witches, hinting at historiographic data, psychological stages, and spiritual hierarchies. By themselves, the magickal formulae are useless, but with the user's ability to meditate on its meaning and internalize it before using it, it becomes powerful.

During rituals and spells, crafted magickal weapons are in use. These weapons help to direct a person's magick. They can also symbolize the user and their psychological elements and metaphysical concepts. Some of the magickal tools witches use include altars, wands, pentacles, swords, daggers, crowns, robes, and lamens. Depending on the user, the meaning these weapons can have can change.

The last commonly used component for ceremonial magick is the vibration of god names. Invocation of deities is very common in ceremonial magick; to do so, users will use a vocal technique known as vibration. Rather than tools, this component is a series of steps, breathing, and thinking patterns. Crowley, a leading teacher of ceremonial magick, described the proper techniques as follows:

> *A physical set of steps, starting in a standing position, breathing in through the nose while imagining the name of the god entering with the breath, imagining that breath traveling through the entire body, stepping forward with the left foot while throwing the body along with arms outstretched, visualizing the name rushing out when spoken, ending in an upright stance, with the right forefinger placed upon the lips (Ceremonial magick, 2021).*

Many Wiccans use this technique in a much simpler version, as they will say the god's name in a drawn-out, long fashion and uses nasal passages, which give the sound and feeling of vibration.

Ceremonial Magick Rituals

Any form of magick that a Wiccan can use has different techniques and purposes and often can be paired with one another. Usually, a witch will employ different types of magick during the same rituals. Then, other witches combine the two to have a more powerful spell. Although the following techniques are said to be ceremonial, they have versions that can be performed with natural magick. It is important to note that how a Wiccan performs the following rituals can differ from clan to clan. There is no set way to practice them.

Banishing

Banishing rituals are performed as a means of eliminating evil, often unseen forces, that are a threat to Wiccans. Often, banishing rituals are used during festivals to protect against fairies and sprites. Remember when we talked about fairies stealing human babies or spirits crossing into the mortal realm to exact revenge? Banishing spells would be used in these situations, along with protection ones. At sabbats, esbats, and other sacred gatherings, many banishing rituals begin the ceremony, ranging from simple to complex practices. Some will rely heavily on natural magick and invoke the elements; others will use the planets, adjacent spaces in astral worlds, or the zodiac signs. But there are limits to banishing rituals as they will not work in an infinite space, so one must be defined with a magick circle or within a singular room.

Purification

Like banishing, purification is typically performed to prepare oneself and space for other spiritual and magickal work. During ancient times, purification was often performed in arduous methods that would last for days, weeks, months, or even lifetimes to remain purified. These purification techniques included sexual abstinence, fasting, diets, excessive cleaning of oneself, and complicated prayers. Although in the present day, these extreme purification practices are no longer used as shorter ones have replaced them. Symbolic purification is also heavily used before ceremonies, including washing oneself and putting on fresh robes.

Consecration

Consecration is a ritual vital to ceremonial magick because it is used to dedicate magickal instruments and spaces for a specific purpose. Wiccans perform consecration rituals on the magickal objects to show their intent and ensure they are not used for dark purposes. Spirits or gods would often be invoked to bless the things as well.

Invocation

Invocation is the act of identifying and bringing forth a spirit or deity. Depending on the Wiccan practices you are using, there are multiple deities or spirits that you could invocate, all of them having different purposes. Crowley and many other Wiccans also believed in the ability to invoke one's secret self or holy guardian angel, which allowed someone to get to know their true selves and their will. There are multiple ways to invoke a deity or spirit, but the magick user must identify with the spirit or deity they are trying to summon. Identifying with the spirit or deity allows for a connection to form, which makes invoking easier. Summoning the spirits of someone you know can be easier because a living link is there; for deities, it can be more challenging because you rely on a spiritual connection, and sometimes gods do not want to answer. However, the same goes for some spirits. They might not want to respond at first.

There are three main categories that invocations can fall into including:

- **Devotion:** This invocation method has someone identifying with the spirit or deity from a place of surrender and love. Users will give up irrelevant and often illusionary parts of themselves that are suppressing them from their full potential.
- **Drama:** Connection with the deity or spirit is created through sympathy and often is invoked through dance or acting. However, this invocation can be complicated as it requires the user to completely lose themselves in their actions and embody the spirit or deity.
- **Calling forth:** The Wiccan using this form, rather than letting go of parts of themselves, will call on their innermost desires, connecting them to the spirit or deity.

Besides the other forms of invocation, assuming the form of a deity or spirit is another option. This entails picturing oneself in the shape of the god or spirit that one wishes to invoke. Each deity represents something, and the user needs to be able to embody this. Typically, Wiccans position themselves in a way associated with the deity or spirit they are trying to summon as if it were enveloping their body. Sometimes, this method also uses the vibration of god names.

Evocation

Invoking and evoking, although they seem alike and perform similar tasks, are quite distinct. Evoking is the act of calling upon a deity, spirit, or entity to request their presence, services, guidance, or knowledge. Hence, the focus is on establishing a connection or communication with the entity and seeking their help or insights. Meanwhile, invoking involves drawing the energy, essence, or presence of a deity or spirit into oneself or a specific space. Subsequently, its purpose is to connect with and merge with the energy or consciousness of the entity to bring about transformation, guidance, inspiration, or spiritual communion. However, not all Wiccans participate in both practices; evoking typically calls upon gods and spirits to supply services or advice. When asking for help, gods are rarely summoned; usually, it is spirits or other entities like demons. Yet, deities can be evoked for information-gathering purposes. It is believed that Wiccans can call forth up to 72 infernal spirits with an evocation ritual that often involves drawing a triangle to give the spirit or god a place to enter.

Eucharist

Originally derived from the word "thanksgiving," Eucharist is now used by Wiccans and other magickal communities to signify the transformation of regular food or drink into holier sacraments. Then, these sacred sacraments are consumed by the coven or an individual. Many kitchen, green, or hearth witches partake in eucharist rituals as they infuse food and drink with magickal properties. Depending on the type of eucharist rituals, the divine properties allow the consumer to embody a deity.

Divination

Divination is used mainly for gathering information and obtaining a guide from the spirit world. It is important to note that divination and fortune-telling are different. Fortune-telling is more about telling the future, while divination is more about looking toward the past and gathering information. Divination is meant to help the Wiccan to gain insight into the decisions they need to make. Many different divinatory techniques can be used based on the type of Wicca or coven you are in. Western Wicca and occult methods of divination include:

- **Astrology:** using divination to learn of the influence heavenly bodies have.
- **Tarot:** the use of a deck of 78 cards, each of which has its meaning, and the user will pick a few cards and determine a message from them.
- **Bibliomancy:** choosing random passages from books and reading them to gain meaning.
- **Geomancy:** the Wiccan will make random marks on the earth or on paper to form 16 patterns and determine meaning from this.

Although divination is accepted, it is not infallible due to the subjectivity of each Wiccan's interpretation.

Ceremonial Magick, the Elementals, and Spirits

Ceremonial magick is renowned for calling upon and summoning spirits, often with the assistance of the elements, to target specific types of entities. Although ceremonial magick does not require the use of the elements, they can be drawn on to help enhance rituals. Each element is associated with a different spirit, and they are as follows:

- **Earth spirits = gnomes:** These spirits are often called upon because of their vast knowledge about the earth's power and locations of riches. They are often called the guardians of earth's treasures as they live underground, guarding them. These spirits embody earthen qualities and are said to be able to dissolve into tree trunks or the ground to hide. Other spirits that are associated with earth include brownies, dryads, earth spirits, elves, pans, and satyrs.
- **Fire spirit = salamander:** Out of all four elements, fire is regarded to be the strongest. Yet, many believe that physical fire could not exist without aid from salamanders. Although no particular species of salamander has been assigned as the spirit of fire, many representations mean that they are around a foot tall or just small-looking balls of lightness or 'sparks.' Salamanders are also believed to reduce in size or amplify themselves and are considered naughty creatures. But much like other spirits, they are influenced by the thinking of humankind and can be dangerous when out of control.
- **Air spirits = sylphs:** These spirits are believed to live at the top of mountains and are changeable and volatile. They also vary in size and work through the winds and gases in their area. While often depicted with wings, they can also be seen in human form. Sylphs have been asso-

ciated with helping humans with creativity, which is why many people will go to high and windy places to work.
- **Water spirit = undines:** These spirits are known to be graceful and beautiful, residing in oceans, waterfalls, and lakes. They take care of the plants growing beneath the surface, displaying a human form, sometimes naked or encased in an almost transparent material similar to water. Sizes can differ depending on their energy levels. And while they may be emotional, they are also said to be friendly.

Ceremonial magick is truly amazing and can be used to learn so much more about the natural world and the unseen world. Embracing your magick, you can learn much more about yourself and the world thanks to ceremonial magick. In the next chapter, we will discuss the third type of magick Wiccans can practice: celestial magick.

11

Celestial Magick

To top off the three types of magick a Wiccan can practice, there is celestial magick. As it sounds, celestial magick deals with the divine. Still, it can be tough to give a concrete definition because depending on the coven or type of Wiccan you have, celestial and the divine can have different meanings and figures. Celestial magick focuses on learning the interactions gods have with mortals and the earth and invoking gods in the hope of causing earthly changes. The beliefs and methods used in celestial magick will change depending on the person performing it. It can be one of the most personal of the three magicks adapting to each user's values. Although it varies based on the user's beliefs, there are a few constants no matter the Wiccan's beliefs or values, which we will discuss throughout this chapter.

Constant 1: Prayer

The first constant in celestial magick is the method in which a Wiccan or other users communicate with deities: prayer. Prayer forms a pseudo-telepathic link, synergy, or emanation, enabling a connection between the Wiccan and the god of their choice. Different prayers might be used for various deities. Often, celestial magic is used to seek guidance, aid, or hand over daily worries and stresses to the gods. But when using it, a person needs to know the specific deity they are trying to communicate with, or they could connect with one that is more sinister or will not be of help. Besides that, celestial magick is also used with special ceremonies to please the spirit being called upon and protect the practitioner from other forces that might cause harm. Some common ceremonial rituals used with celestial magick include purification, offerings, blessings, sanctification, and asking for favors. However, there is still a high chance of failure when attempting to ask an entity to stop doing something, which can result in the anger of deities with unforeseen consequences, something Wiccans do not want to risk.

Constant 2: Spirituality

Celestial magic's second tenet is the spiritual nature of the divine, to whom Wiccans pray instead of one another. These Wiccans are considered heavenly because their prayers are directed towards non-physical beings with power and intelligence over the earth, such as stellar, ethereal, infernal, or celestial. Among other divine beings, astral deities are the only one that lives amongst the stars. Meanwhile, other spirits that can be called upon often live in an undefined space or multiple plains as their importance, meaning, or influence shifts. As we learned earlier in this book, the Horned God changes locations throughout the year to signify the different seasons.

Though summoning and celestial magic may appear the same, there is a notable contrast between them: the type of spirit involved and the power of the Wiccan. While performing a summoning ritual, the Wiccan controls the spirit. If something starts to go wrong, the Wiccan can maintain control and send the spirit back to where it came from. But in celestial magick, the Wiccan cannot act arrogant, restrict, nor control the deity they communicate with. Instead, they must be humble in asking for help or guidance, as demanding something of a deity will only anger them.

Constant 3: Workings of Celestial Magick

The third constant of celestial magick is the skills and abilities which celestial Wiccans need to have knowledge and practice. One of the essential skills that Wiccans need to perform celestial magick is divine intervention. Although more mundane or inhuman spirits are not assumed to have high levels of intelligence, deities allow celestial Wiccans to ask them to complete much larger goals rather than a simple task or two. Giving the care of problems into the hands of the deity can ensure they are done faster, and the Wiccan no longer needs to worry about something. Depending on the problem, deities can also be sure to check up on situations and keep the coven safe.

Another skill that celestial Wiccans have is protection from deities. If a celestial Wiccan feels that they are in trouble or that their coven is in grave danger, they can seek the protection of a deity. Many deities use the world's energies to make changes that the celestial Wiccans have asked of them. Deities can also adapt to circumstances and observe situations, making decisions based on what is happening. However, it is important to remember that a deity is not bound to listen to you, and although your goals might be met, they might not be as you thought they would be.

The third skill that these witches have is overpowering lesser spirits. Not all Wiccans can conquer lesser spirits, which is why celestial Wiccans and their abilities can be of great value to a coven. A celestial Wiccan can ask for a deity to lend them their strength, which can help them to vanquish demons or dispel troublesome spirits. However, a deity must be willing to give some of its power to the user.

Celestial magick can be one of a coven's most advantageous powers, often with the leader seeking this magick to protect the coven from danger. The intelligence of the deities can be a great tool as they have lived much longer and experienced much more than the person. However, celestial Wiccans must tread lightly because not all deities are friendly or willing to help. Now that you know the three types of magick that Wiccans can use, it is time to move on to the fifth and final pillar: rituals.

Pillar 5
Rituals

Rituals have been part of the Wiccan tradition for centuries, providing structure and guidance to those who practice their faith. In this chapter, we will explore some of the common components found in rituals, and different types of altars, tools, and ritual wear used when performing these ceremonies.

We will begin by looking at altars—what they are, what items you typically find on them, and where you should locate them in a room and decorate it. Then, we will also discuss the various tools that make up a witch's arsenal, from the pentacle to the cauldron, and how they function within a ritual. Finally, we will examine which clothing fits a Wiccan ceremony and how a ritual is properly carried out from start to finish.

Once we have gone through all these topics, you will better understand the rich symbolism behind each component of ritual work and be ready to apply them in your journey as an individual or with others around you. So, let us dive into this fascinating topic and discover more about the rituals of Wiccans!

12

Altars

Various components go into a single ritual or spell, the first being the altar. Altars are a common element among different belief systems, including Wicca. The altar used can have different purposes, but most rituals will have some form of altar. For Wiccans, the primary use of an altar is to be a physical structure meant to honor deities, ancestors, and other spirits, or they are also meant to hold the ritual object that will be used. Altars also serve as the focal point of celebrations, so an altar will be in the center of one of the eight sabbats, esbats, or any other celebration that a Wiccan might have. For covens, this might be a permanent altar in the center of the coven grounds. There are also often small altars inside witches' homes, or they will make them perform spells in the house. Throughout this chapter, we will discuss the typical Wiccan altar and various ways you can set one up.

The Wiccan Altar

Depending on the type of Wiccan a person is, the look and location of an altar can vary. Altars belonging to covens may be located outdoors, in a designated building, or within the leader's home, which is used for rituals with the entire coven. Furthermore, many spells are based on particular locations, prompting Wiccans to have small altars in their houses.

Variations in the appearance of a Wiccan altar also depend on the available space. For solitary Wiccans with limited space, a double-duty altar is ideal as it allows them to use it for rituals, spells, and regular activities. Often, double-duty altars are kept in small sizes that can be neatly tucked away when not in use. Desks and tables work best for this purpose. As regards its shape, it is entirely up to the Wiccan and their space. Yet, most Wiccans prefer circle-shaped as it allows movement while mimicking the sacred circle made before rituals. Natural materials, such as wood or stone, are also chosen because they can connect a Wiccan to nature, especially if they do not have access. And so willow and oak are often selected for altars.

Transforming a space in your house into an altar can be done by performing rituals that imbue it with magickal energy. This is particularly helpful for future ceremonies and spells you may wish to do. Meanwhile, wood and other natural products are recommended, as nature typically holds more power for magickal practices. As you get closer to nature, the more potent the outcome of your rituals and spells will be. But if you have access to a natural area that provides security, feel free to use a large stump or flat rock as an altar.

Types of Altars

Different altars can affect the power of your rituals and spells. With so many options, the type you have can make a difference. Yet, altars that contain more natural products are more powerful than those made of artificial products. Here are some different kinds of altars you can create, especially if you do not have access to natural spaces.

Box Shrine

These shrines are relatively small and can be designed to honor a singular god, goddess, or deity. Often, these shrines or altars are created in suitcases, which can be great if you are trying to connect to a past relative with some connection to the briefcase. However, not all carry-ons are made with natural material, so if you are planning to make this kind of altar, having links to other Wiccans, such as a relative, can give it the little boost of power that it needs. These altars are also transportable, which is a nice feature if you travel somewhere to perform the rituals. Also, if you do not feel safe having your altar open when people visit, this form allows you to close it up and out of sight.

Shrine

Unlike traditional box shrines, Wiccan shrines are typically fixed in a dedicated room for rituals and prayer. The complexity, ranging from simple to extravagant, is entirely up to you. Besides, anything from a simple to an elaborate shrine altar can be used as a point of focus to revere a god, goddess, spirit, or deity. To create one, you need items representing what you worship, relevant tools such as incense or centers, and decorations. Flowers or natural objects can also add the right touch of nature if the shrine is crafted from non-natural material like plastic.

Adding more objects to the altar or shrine will make it more susceptible to magick. And if you have a specific purpose for a ritual, you can add crystals, herbs, and candles. There are often occasions in which a Wiccan decorate their altar more heavily. Samhain, or the beginning of the Wiccan year, and the time in which the veil between the spirit and human world is thinnest, make their altars or shrines much more elaborate, such as with lots of pictures of passed family members. Some also move the shrine to the central area of the house so that the entire family can get together and feast. But other people only decorate their altars decorated during sabbats or other celebrations.

Tabletop Altar

Tabletop altars are just as they sound; they are made on the top of a table. Many people hosting rituals in their homes may create a temporary altar on the top of a table in a big room for the entire group. These altars are also often made when someone has a shrine that cannot be moved, but they want the ritual celebration to be in another house room that is more fitting.

Ritual Altar

Ritual altars are typically the most complicated to construct, as they are designed for meaningful rituals during sabbats and esbats. Essentially, they require a wide range of tools, including a wand, athame, pentagram, candles, incense, and any other objects you may need for a ritual. Due to their size, usually much larger than regular permanent altars, it requires more space to arrange all the elements correctly.

Working Altar

Not all altars are built for magickal rituals; some exist to honor gods or loved ones. Prayers can be said at these altars, but no magickal practices may occur there. Working altars, however, are those that are made to carry out magick-related tasks. Likewise, these altars should be kept uncluttered and contain only the necessary objects so the magick can avoid accidentally diverting them elsewhere. Also, make sure you customize your altar suited to your abilities and the rituals and spells you plan to work with. And remember, altars set up for daily magick differ from those meant for sabbats, esbats, and celebrations as they are more simplistic yet effective. Meanwhile, festivity altars require more elements to be included in them due to the complexity of their purpose.

Often, a witch can have multiple altars that serve different purposes. They can have one for magickal rituals and spells, one for prayer and honoring deities or spirits, and another for rituals performed during sabbats and esbats.

Setting up An Altar

Depending on which type of altar you are putting together, there are plenty of ways to craft one, but let us assume that you are making an altar on a piece of furniture you already own. To start, cover the altar with fabrics or scarves of different colors. When deciding on the colors for your ritual, you may choose meaningful shades or whatever's easiest to find if you are in a pinch. Many people often change the fabrics with the seasons to mimic the year cycle. Depending on the ritual being performed, different textiles might be used. The decorations might also go through the same changes as the fabric. Still, it is entirely up to the Wiccan who decorate the altar. An example of decoration you might see being rotated is holly berries and fir leaves during Yule. On top of seasonal or ritual decorations, you can use your favorite crystals, stones, images of deities, or any other item.

When deciding on a layout for your altar, you have many options. Some are more intricate, while others are quite simple—it all depends on your performing ritual. But generally speaking, the altar is split down the middle. The left side represents the Triple Goddess and has tools that align with her and the elements of earth and water. While on the right side symbolizes the Horned God and includes those tools associated with him and the elements of fire and air

Another layout has objects meant to represent the Triple Goddess and the Horned God in the center of the altar and the tools required for the ritual in order of element: earth in the north, the air in the east, fire in the south, and water in the west.

Some Wiccans also decorate their altars eclectically, which means they intuitively decorate the altar, allowing their consciousness to find patterns and places they resonate with. But whether it is elaborate or basic, how you design your altar is totally up to you. The amount of space available also plays a huge role in arranging it. Thus, your options may be more restricted if there is little space.

Where to set up your altar is totally up to you. Pick the spot that feels right, even if it is inside your home, outside, or anywhere you feel connected. And if you have a grimoire that outlines specific directions on constructing an altar for particular rituals, you may follow those instructions. But you could also follow your intuition if it does not provide further direction. After you set up your altar, it is time to gather all the tools you will need to participate in your rituals and spells, which we will learn about in the next chapter.

13

Tools

Setting up the altar can be considered laying the foundations for your ritual, and now it is time to start building up that foundation using various tools. However, remember that not all magick requires magickal tools, and not all tools will be used during a ritual. Natural magick very rarely uses artificial tools but relies on nature. Some rituals in natural magick, especially more extensive rituals performed by covens, use tools to help direct the magick. Meanwhile, ceremonial and celestial magick depend on them much more heavily. Yet, tools are not always used to direct magick; they are often used to honor gods, goddesses, or deities. Here are the most commonly used magickal tools and items used by Wiccans.

Pentacle

A pentacle is a consecration tool that is placed on an altar. Typically, pentacles have a magickal symbol or sigil engraved on them. Although the emblem engraved on them might be different for some Wiccans, it is commonly a circle with a pentagram inside. The pentacle symbolizes the earth element, often used for evoking blessings and energizing items. Likewise, it acts as an indicator of things that have been blessed and provides a means to charge them up with spiritual power.

Pentacles are the most commonly used tools in almost any ritual or spell a Wiccan might perform. They can be made from any material, including clay, wood, metal, or wax. But the more natural the material, the better, as it will be easier to infuse with magickal abilities. In ceremonial magick, pentacles serve as protective talismans. Creating your pentacle can be an empowering experience, allowing you to pour your magick and energy into it in a way you would not be able to with a purchased one. But if making one is not an option, plenty of ready-made versions are available.

Sword or Knife

Ritual swords or knives, known as athames, are utilized in Wiccan rituals, with Gardnerian Wicca highly dependent on them as they represent the element of fire. These double-edged daggers usually come with a black handle, sometimes decorated with etchings. Wiccans can also opt for either crafting or purchasing their athames. But it is important to note that they are rarely used for cutting or directing magick. And for many Wiccans, using an athame to draw blood is seen as defiling the tool, so it usually needs to be destroyed afterward.

Wand

Wands can take many forms, with some representing fire and others symbolizing air. But Gardnerian Wicca holds to the latter. Materials used to make wands range from rock and wood to metal and even crystals. To further personalize their wand, they may add engravings of runes, stones, or crystals that are meaningful to them. For many practitioners of natural magic, wands can be a helpful tool for amplifying and channeling their energy. These can be made more effective by adding crystals to the wand. However, not all crystals are suitable for embedding into wands.

Having a dual purpose, wands direct magick and energy and summon spirits. In many Wiccan traditions, these methods are interchangeable. Meanwhile, fairies and other elemental spirits were historically said to be scared of iron and steel, so wands made from natural materials are generally preferred for summoning. In contrast, metal ones are employed for containment. Although athames can sometimes serve the same purpose, wands are still considered stronger and more suitable for handling spirits. Typically, witches who do not rely on athames resort to using a wand for summoning.

Furthermore, wands are a phallic symbol representing male power, virility, and energy. Rituals for the Horned God will often have wands in them to honor him. Invoking deities and consecrating spaces are also performed using wands.

Chalice

Chalices or goblets are cups used to represent the element of water. In some traditions, the chalice is not used as a tool but as a representation of the Triple Goddess' womb. But even during rituals that are not exclusive to the Triple Goddess, a chalice or cauldron is typically present to symbolize the feminine energy and representation of a womb. Likewise, at symbolic rituals of the Great Rite, chalices and athames stand for femininity. Some popular materials for these items include pewter and silver.

Boline

Bolines are another type of knife that can be used during rituals. These knives traditionally have a white handle and a curved blade in the shape of a crescent moon. Unlike the athame, bolines have practical uses, including cutting herbs, harvesting crops, inscribing candles with sigils or symbols, and cutting ritual cords.

Although these tools might not be used during the actual ritual, they are used for physical preparation. Moreover, they represent two distinct realms: the human plane and the spiritual plane. For the physical plane, bolines are used, while athames are for the spiritual one.

Censer and Incense

Burning incense is a common practice to create a calming atmosphere, especially during religious ceremonies. Different fragrances can evoke the gods, goddesses, and deities associated with different times of the year. Furthermore, censers are containers that hold and release incense smoke during prayer.

Besom

Besoms, a term for a broom, is used to clean out ceremonial spaces before a ritual is performed. By sweeping, the Wiccan who does this duty removes the negative energy. And so before a ritual, it is essential to clean away negative energies that can otherwise affect the outcome. This purifying tool is connected to the element of water, and besoms, like wands, are phallic symbols often used in fertility dances. During handfasting ceremonies, a couple will also jump over a besom as part of the ritual.

Cauldron

When witches come to mind, two of the first images likely to appear are a besom and wands. The third image commonly associated with witches is a cauldron, which can be used in place of a chalice, particularly in female-oriented rituals. Cauldrons are seen as feminine and symbolic of water, making them an essential part of many rituals and often placed on an altar filled with liquid. Plus, it has relevance in honoring the Triple Goddess in feminine-focused rites. Meanwhile, in Celtic mythology and tradition, cauldrons are associated with the goddess Cerridwen, who has prophetic abilities and is the cauldron keeper of inspiration and knowledge and resides in the underworld.

Cauldrons have numerous magickal uses, including burning offerings, incense, and candles, blending herbs, representation of the Triple Goddess or any other goddesses, and using for moonlight scrying when filled with water. Using a cauldron for culinary purposes is not recommended, as the primary purpose of a cauldron is for practicing magick. Rather than cooking, a cauldron is better utilized in rituals and spells. But if you want to prepare food in a cauldron, have one for magickal purposes and one for food. Often, kitchen witches have multiple cauldrons, but it is essential to remember that cast iron cauldrons intended for cooking must be adequately seasoned.

Spear or Staff

Seax-Wicca tradition uses a spear to represent the god Woden, who takes the place of the Horned God. While not all Wiccans use a spear, their uses of one can differ. In contrast, the staff is more regularly incorporated into Wiccan practices. Although the staff is not essential for Wiccans, many use it to symbolize their authority and power. Representations differ based on culture, but men are often represented by staff. In some, they convey air; in others, fire. When in a coven, the high priest or priestess will carry a staff as a physical embodiment of their power.

Bell

According to folklore, intense noise, such as bells, is thought to ward off evil spirits. So, to keep malicious spirits away, witches often hung bells around their homes and utilized them in outdoor rituals. In particular, witches hoped to repel mischievous entities by ringing bells during outside ceremonies. Likewise, the vibrations caused by bells are often believed to be a power source. Other than bells, you can also use a ritual rattle, sistrum, or singing bowl. The sounds of these tools are also thought to bring harmony during ceremonies.

Candles

Candles are a popular tool for Witches, representing the element of fire. They can be carved and shaped into figures to pay honor to gods or goddesses. Although sometimes used in rituals, they are most frequent in casting spells, as it is said that these objects accumulate one's energy. And once lit, this stored energy combined with magick is released as its flame burns away.

Many Wiccans prefer to make their candles for ritual and spellwork since they believe this increases the item's magickal power. Moreover, crafting a candle can be both a spiritual and an empowering experience as it allows you to pour your energy, magickal abilities, and intentions into its creation. Yet, other Wiccans believe that making a candle does not make a difference; the intent behind burning a candle is what gives it more power. Different colors and aromas are also often used in rituals and ceremonies throughout the year, each having a special meaning and purpose.

Crystals

As we have learned in previous chapters throughout this book, crystals are very common in Wiccan traditions, no matter the type of Wiccan you might be. Natural magick uses crystals often; however, they are also used in other magick and many Wiccan traditions. Different traditions also use various crystals, and which ones you choose are essential because they represent different elements and attributes. When selecting a new crystal or stone, purify it before you use it for magickal rituals and spells.

Divination Tools

Not all Wiccans use divination. However, those that do have specific tools designed exclusively for clairvoyance. There are many different divination tools, but having only one or two items is all you need. There is also no need to keep them on your altar constantly. But one of the most commonly used divination tools is tarot cards.

Remember, you do not need to pile on every tool under the sun when performing a ritual, nor do they not all necessarily have to be present on your altar. Use only the tools necessary, and there is no need to overdo it. Hence, if you do not need any staff for a ritual, there is no point in having them around. But now that you have your altar and what you need, the next aspect of a ceremony you need to have is your ritual wear, which we will discuss in the next chapter.

14

Ritual Wear

What a Wiccan chooses to wear for their ritual is solely up to them. Although, many traditions could be followed from the practices of witches, which were said to have inspired the practices of Wicca. During its beginnings, it was popular for those taking part in rituals to go skyclad or even nude. However, for modern Wicca, this is rarely how people conduct rituals. Depending on whether you are part of a coven or practicing solitarily, the ritual wear you have might differ. In a coven, different attire might be required for ritual practice. But if you practice alone, it is your choice whether to stick with tradition. Here are some of the most commonly worn ritual wear that Wiccans use.

Ritual Robes

Taking on a robe is more than just putting on the physical garment; it is about preparing for the ritual, embracing ancient customs, and connecting with those who have come before. The primary purpose of wearing ritual robes is to distinguish oneself from the mundane and enhance your magick. Many take a cleansing bath before donning their ritual robes to ensure they are as pure as possible. Traditionally, Wiccan robes should go without anything else underneath, allowing one to embody their nature fully; however, this is your choice.

For those in a coven, the color of their robe can indicate their rank within the group. However, not all covens are like this. Likewise, if you are practicing solitarily, you can have multiple robes of different styles and colors for specific rituals or during different seasons. Colors that are associated with each season include blue (spring), green (summer), brown (fall), and white (winter). Usually, many Wiccans opt for white or earthy tones to harmonize with nature and avoid black due to its negative symbolism. Despite this, you do not need to feel obliged to stick to traditional seasonal fabrics, but still, pay attention to the type of fabric and color you wear.

When crafting or purchasing a robe, one thing to bear in mind is the presence of candles and fire during rituals. Due to this, having a robe made of materials that cannot catch fire is essential for safety. The design of your robe can also be as intricate or simple as you prefer.

Wiccans who create their robe put in the extra effort to make them meaningful by customizing and filling them with their energy and magickal abilities. But even for those inexperienced with sewing, creating a robe is doable, as patterns are available in-store and online. For a good design in stores, look for one under costumes. Historical and Renaissance are also categories you can look for robes. Here are sewing patterns you can find online that are perfect for creating ritual robes:

- **Simplicity 4795**: For those participating in a passion play, an angel-designed ritual robe is an ideal choice for Wiccans. Although slight alterations to the sleeve length might be needed, it is an easy pattern for beginners to follow.
- **Simplicity 3616:** Though it is a campy wizard costume, the robe is perfect for a masculine version of a ritual robe. Just be sure to discard the long white beard and trim.

- **Simplicity 3623:** This is a Scottish-themed costume with a masculine underdress under the skirt and bodice and an uncomplicated pattern that works well for a ceremonial robe.

These three patterns are all beginner friendly and simple. But if you want a more elaborate robe and are an advanced sewer, try the McCall 4490; it is a perfect Renaissance-style dress that can be used as a ritual robe.

Buying a pattern is not necessary, either. You can make one without it. There are a few supplies that you will need, including a sewing machine, six feet of cord or light rope, measuring tape, scissors, thread, your fabric of choice, and tailor's chalk. Follow these steps to make a robe without a pattern:

1. Get help from another person to take your measurements properly. Outstretch your arms and measure the length from wrist to wrist. Write this measurement down with the letter "A" next to it.
2. Measure the distance between the nape of your neck to the area even with your ankle, and write this down with the letter "B."
3. Fold your material in half and cut out a T shape using the measurements you got for "A" and "B." Do not cut along the fold.
4. Measure out the center of measurement "A" and cut a hole for your head. Make sure it is not too large or will slide off your shoulders.
5. Sew on the underside of the arm, leaving the end of the T open for hands. Sew from the armpit to the bottom. Turn the robe inside right, trying it on to make adjustments.
6. Add a cord around the waist. If you are practicing solitarily, you can create this cord for yourself. Depending on whether you are in a coven, this cord might be provided

to you at initiation and as you progress through different levels of training.

7. If you would like, add trim, beading, and other designs to the robe to make it more personal. Magickal symbols can also be sewn into robes.
8. Before wearing your robe, be sure to purify it.

Cloaks

Cloaks can be crafted or purchased. And since they do not provide sufficient body coverage with only a clasp, ties, or button at the neck, they are commonly worn over a robe during colder months. Yet, some more lavish versions do come with hoods and sleeves attached. However, sometimes you do not need a cloak if the ritual takes place indoors.

For both cloaks and robes, there is no need to go out and buy an expensive one. You can use clothing you already have and remake them into a robe or cloak. If your family practices Wicca, you can use their cloaks and robes.

Pentacle

We talked about pentacles in the last chapter because they are a common tool used by Wiccans. To recap, pentacles are a consecration tool and often hold blessed items. When placed on an altar, they are usually made of stone, wood, clay, metal, or other natural materials. There are several ways to wear a pentacle, including jewelry or sewing it into your garments.

When performing rituals or evocation, identifying yourself as a Wiccan can be essential for the deities you are trying to summon. Wearing a pentacle on your person during rituals is a way of declaring yourself as a Wiccan. However, during specific times, such as Samhain, wearing any markers of you being a Wiccan should be avoided because it will attract spirits and fairies that want to try to play tricks on you.

Other Jewelry

There is no specific jewelry that a Wiccan must wear; this is a highly personal part of the ritual wear of Wiccans. In covens, it might be required not to wear jewelry, so they are as close to sky-clad as possible while wearing a robe. Any jewelry worn during rituals is typically magickal, containing runes or symbols that are meaningful to the person. Yet, some ritual jewelry may differ as each can boost the spell's power and Wiccan's abilities. Any jewelry that enhances one's energy can be worn during a ceremony.

Many Wiccans also craft special pieces with crystals they feel connected to, wearing them in everyday life and during rituals to benefit from them. Meanwhile, others may opt to create jewelry honoring gods or deities. But it is an entirely personal process. If you are out and shopping for jewelry, focus on how you feel when you pick a piece. For such, when you touch a piece of jewelry and feel a buzz of energy, that is a sign that this is for you and is boosting your energy.

Overall, what you wear during a ritual is very personal, especially when practicing solitarily. Although it is best to wear a robe during ceremonies, there are no strict rules. Aside from that, you can also make your robes, cloaks, and jewelry personal, boosting your energy. We have the altar, the tools, and the ritual wear you need, and now it is time to explore the standard components of a Wiccan ritual.

15

Common Components of Wiccan Rituals

Depending on the type of Wicca you practice, how rituals are performed can differ, but the bare bones of a ritual, no matter the form of Wicca you practice, are similar. Think back to celestial magick and the commonalities it has, despite there being so many different types. The same goes for Wiccan rituals. Many types of ceremonies can be performed, and each kind of Wicca can do them differently. There are several types of rituals and spells that Wiccans can perform, and they have different purposes and meanings. We will learn more about the kinds of rituals in the next chapter, but first, let us know the essential components that all Wiccan rituals have.

Preparation

Before starting any spell or ritual, preparation is necessary. For spells, a witch may need to have their ingredients and tools ready. Consecrating those tools, garments, and even the Wiccan is essential for a successful ritual. Neglecting proper preparation can have a serious impact on ritual success as well as one's ability to cast magick.

The primary purposes of consecration are to purify objects used in the ceremony and to cleanse them of any dark energy that could have gathered. This is essential, as these tools must interact with the Divine, and if there is dark energy, it can damage rituals. As with an empty room, unwanted energy can accumulate over time, like dust, so it is essential to clear it out before performing any new ritual. Hence, this is why consecration must always take place between practices.

Although consecrating your tools before a ritual is optional, it is still a great practice to develop, especially if you use a pre-owned tool. With consecration, it is also possible to know what types of energies have been used or what kind of magick has been performed with your tool. Likewise, before using any brand-new tools, purify them once. After that, performing a consecration occasionally should be enough for upkeep.

How often you choose to consecrate your tools is entirely up to you. Yet, it would be best to do it as often as possible to ensure dark magick or energy is not messing with your rituals. You can also cleanse the space where your altar and tool are to reduce how much consecration you need to do.

Different people may perform a consecration differently. And as there are many variations in this process, one thing remains the same: getting to know the four elements is an integral part of the ritual. When performing a consecration, there is no wrong or right way to do it as long as the tool is connected with the four elements. So, your ceremony can be as detailed or minimalistic as you would like. Once the four elements have blessed the tool, it is considered purified.

For the consecration ceremony, you will need a cup of water, a white candle, a small bowl of salt, and incense. Each of these items represents a direction and an element:

- Salt (north and earth)
- Incense (east and air)
- Candle (south and fire)
- Water (west and water)

At this point, some Wiccans will cast a circle before their consecration, but this is not necessary. After you have gathered the materials and have your tools, cast the circle if you decide to. Place each of the items in their proper spot and light the candle and incense. Here is an example of how you might perform the consecration.

Grab the tool you are consecrating, and start by facing north. Pass the item over the salt and say the following words:

> *"Powers of the North,*
> *Guardians of the Earth,*
> *I consecrate this wand of willow (or knife of steel, amulet of crystal, etc.)*
> *and charge it with your energies.*
> *I purify it this night and make this tool sacred" (Wigington, 2019a).*

Turn to face the east, and pass the item or tool through the smoke of the incense and say the words:

> *"Powers of the East,*
> *Guardians of the Air,*
> *I consecrate this wand of willow*
> *and charge it with your energies.*
> *I purify it this night and make this tool sacred" (Wigington, 2019a).*

Face the south and pass the item over the fire. Be extra cautious here because many items are flammable. Say these words as you pass the item over the fire:

"Powers of the South,
Guardians of Fire,
I consecrate this wand of willow
and charge it with your energies.
I purify it this night and make this tool sacred" (Wigington, 2019a).

Turn to face west and pass the item over the water, saying the words:

"Powers of the West,
Guardians of Water,
I consecrate this wand of willow [or knife of steel, amulet of crystal, etc.]
and charge it with your energies.
I purify it this night and make this tool sacred" (Wigington, 2019a).

Last, face the altar and hold your item up to the sky and say the following words:

"I charge this wand in the name of Old Ones,
the Ancients, the Sun and the Moon, and the Stars.
By the powers of the Earth, of Air, of Fire, and Water
I banish the energies of any previous owners
and make it new and fresh.
I consecrate this wand,
and it is mine." (Wigington, 2019a).

Taking a shower before dressing in your gown is an excellent method to consecrate the person. This consecration ritual being performed is mainly for tools. Consecrating your robes can also occur in this manner, but avoid getting the garment too close to the candle's fire.

In some Wiccan traditions, some will immediately use their recently consecrated tool to bind it. Using the newly purified tool in a ritual right after is also believed to increase its strength.

Casting the Magick Circle

Depending on the ceremony and tradition, you might cast a magick circle before consecration or after. There is no right or wrong way of doing it. Magick circles are performed before every ritual, whether you are in a coven or not. Although casting a magick circle is not absolute, there are no definite rules that need to be followed for witchcraft; however, casting a magick circle can help boost your magick's power and ward off evil spirits and energy while you are working.

Just as with the consecration ritual, there are multiple ways to cast a magick circle that can change based on what tools and materials you have on hand or how much time you have. You will not need to do an elaborate magick circle for quick rituals, but a simple one. Many people use four candles to represent the direction and chant as they light each one. A person might also include an item representing the four seasons and elements, but this is unnecessary. In the sample casting of a magick circle I share with you, you will have different colored candles symbolizing the elements.

To cast a magick circle, you will need the following:

- A besom
- A green candle to represent the north
- A yellow candle to represent the east
- A red candle to represent the south

- A blue candle to represent the west
- Incense
- Salt, pine branches, or flowers
- Bowl of water
- Bowl of salt

Cleanse the area you are performing your ritual with a besom first. This way, you will rid the area of any dark energy that has gathered since the last ritual you had. Once you have cleansed the room, it is time to set up the candles, starting in the north. Set each candle up, going clockwise. If performing some form of dark magick, you will go counterclockwise.

Depending on the type of ritual, you will either have the candles inside the circle or outside of it, as we talked about in an earlier chapter. Ensure that your altar is inside the circle. Have a bowl of salt and water on the altar as well. Light incense and candles before grabbing your wand or athame from the altar and place the point at the bowl of water and say,

> *"I consecrate and cleanse this water so it may be purified and fit to dwell within the sacred circle.*
>
> *In the name of the Mother Goddess and the Father God [or the names of specific deities], I consecrate this water" (How to Cast a Wicca Ritual Magick Circle, 2021).*

When you say these words, imagine you are blasting away all the negative energy that might be contained in the water. Move the point of your dagger or wand to touch the bowl of salt and say:

> *"I bless this salt that it may be fit to dwell within the sacred circle.*

> *In the name of the Mother Goddess and the Father God, I bless this salt" (How to Cast a Wicca Ritual Magick Circle, 2021).*

After blessing the water and salt, hold your athame or wand at waist height and slowly walk around the circle clockwise. As you walk around the circle, charge it with your magick energy. Imagine your energy stretching and forming a sphere, half above the ground and half underground. Remember that spirits and otherworldly beings can appear from anywhere, including beneath. Say these words as you walk around the circle:

> *"Here is the boundary of the circle.*
> *Naught but love shall enter in.*
> *Naught but love shall emerge from within.*
> *Charge this by your powers, Old Ones!" (How to Cast a Wicca Ritual Magick Circle, 2021).*

Take the salt and sprinkle it to form a circle, starting and ending in the north. If you are using flowers or branches, place them to form a circle. Repeat the process with the incense and water, sprinkling it around the circle's parameter. At this point, the circle is sealed, but you can take it further if you wish.

The circle is now complete, and with the spirits of the elements invoked, it helps to grow your power, and you can now perform any spell or ritual or evoke or invoke any deity you would like.

Calling the Quarters and Invoking the Deities

Calling the quarters goes by many names, including calling the elements or the guardians of the watchtowers. This ritual can be viewed as a supplement to the casting of a magick circle; invoking the four elements and spirits is used to amplify the power of this kind of secret circle. Getting in touch with the quarters or invoking deities can be done without a specific method. Everyone is free to choose the most meaningful and powerful approach; there's no one right way. Besides, all you need is an athame or wand, nothing else. Still, if you would like, you can also put a tool associated with each element in the appropriate cardinal direction, marked by the candles you used for casting the magick circle.

Once you have placed each of the tools, if you choose to, in each cardinal direction, it is time to start summoning the spirits. There are numerous ways to imagine the elements and their spirits. You might imagine the spirit forms we discussed earlier in the book or just an embodiment of the element. Either will work.

Holding your wand or athame toward the north, imagine a green mist rising from the candle, forming a spirit or trees, and say the words:

> *"O Spirit of the North,*
> *Ancient One of Earth,*
> *I call you to attend this circle.*
> *Charge this by your powers, Old Ones!" (How to Cast a Wicca Ritual Magick Circle, 2021).*

Move to the east, visualizing a yellow mist becoming a spirit or whirlwind, and say the words:

> *"O Spirit of the East,*
> *Ancient One of Air,*
> *I call you to attend this circle.*
> *Charge this by your powers, Old Ones!" (How to Cast a Wicca Ritual Magick Circle, 2021).*

Move to the south, visualizing a red mist becoming a spirit or flames, and say the words:

> *"O Spirit of the South,*
> *Ancient One of Fire,*
> *I call you to attend this circle.*
> *Charge this by your powers, Old Ones!" (How to Cast a Wicca Ritual Magick Circle, 2021).*

Last, move to the west, visualizing a blue mist becoming a spirit or wave, and repeat the words:

> *"O Spirit of the West,*
> *Ancient One of Water,*
> *I call you to attend this circle.*
> *Charge this by your powers, Old Ones!" (How to Cast a Wicca Ritual Magick Circle, 2021).*

Visualization is key to calling the quarters or summoning a deity because you have to connect with them. They are in the spiritual plane, so you must use your third eye and visualization skills to make the initial connection. Your power will then help to form the connection. For specific deities, there will be different ways to summon them. Symbols and different words might be used for other deities. If you have a grimoire, it will likely outline the different ways your specific Wiccan type invokes or evokes a deity.

The Heart of the Ritual and the Book of Shadows

After you have prepared the ritual, cast the circle, and summoned the element, spirits, or deities you need, it is time for the heart of the ritual, which will be the main ritual you want to perform. You can do various things, including grounding, centering, or shielding, which we will learn about in the next chapter.

The Book of Shadows is a sacred text for all Wiccans, but not all Wiccans have access to it. This book is said to contain instructions for many magickal rituals. Many grimoires that Wiccans come across were derived from the Book of Shadows. Gerald Gardner wrote the first and most famous Book of Shadows, which initiated the craft in the 1950s. Although he was the first person to write the book, he allowed others to copy it and change it to fit their needs better. It was believed that a Book of Shadows would work for only the owner. That is why when other Wiccans read Gerald's version and tried to use the same spells, not all of them worked. They needed to be changed to fit the user better. So, new spells are created, and existing rituals are modified when needed, showing no fixed and rigid way of executing magic. This flexibility allows for much more freedom in practice rather than a restrictive approach.

However, not all Wiccans have access to a Book of Shadows, and it is often believed that there were two versions, one for covens and one for personal use. The personal version of the Book of Shadows will be different for everyone and have various spells, rituals, and recipes.

Eclectic witches have different meanings when it comes to the Book of Shadows. To them, it is a personal journal, not a traditional text. In this journal, a witch would record the result of spells and rituals, how they worked or did not, and any other magickal information they came across during their lifetime. While a Book of Shadows to other witches might be passed on from teacher to student, or copies made for covens, for eclectic witches, they were not typically passed on. An eclectic witch must learn, discover their magick, and create rituals.

Cake and Ale

Throughout many religions, it is a common and sacred act to share food and drinks during different rituals and ceremonies. The same goes for Wiccans. If you practice in a coven or solitary, you will offer ale and cakes to the gods and goddesses and eat them yourself. All participating members would consume the cake and ale in a coven during the ceremony.

Before the casting of the magick circle, cake and ale are prepared and placed on the altar. A chalice will hold the ale being served, and a special plate is often used for the cake to sit on. These dishes are to be used for the cakes and ale alone and for no other purpose, as they could corrupt the food or magick. There is no specific type of cake or ale that is served. Consecration occurs on the cake and ale before being offered. Some people consecrate the food with the tools, while others do it right before offering it to the gods. But be sure to offer the food to the gods before handing it out to everyone else and eating it yourself. Remember, consuming ale and cake without offering some of it to the deity is considered disrespectful by Wiccans.

Closing the Ritual

We are now at the end of the ritual, and although you will always have a connection to the deities you invoked, you have to revoke them, allowing them to leave the circle. Use these words or something similar to revoke a spirit or ritual:

> *"Lady of the Moon, of the fertile Earth and rolling seas,*
> *Lord of the Sun, of the sky and wild,*
> *Thank You for Your presence in our circle today.*
> *Stay if you will, go if you must,*
> *But know that you are ever welcome in our hearts.*
> *We bid you hail and farewell" (Wright, 2022b).*

After you have revoked the deity, goddess, or god you have summoned, you must also revoke the elements. When invoking, we started in the north, but to revoke, you will begin in the west and work counterclockwise. Use your hands, athame, or wand, standing westward, and say:

"Powers of the West: powers of Water;
Thank You for Your presence in our circle today,
For sharing your deep mysteries and intuition,
Hail and farewell, powers of the West" (Wright, 2022b).

Turn toward the south and say:

"Powers in the South; Powers of Fire;
Thank You for Your presence in our circle today,
For sharing your inspiration and courage,
Hail and farewell, powers of the South" (Wright, 2022b).

Turn to the east and say:

"Powers of the East; powers of Earth,
Thank you for Your presence in our circle today;
For sharing your stability and growth,
Hail and farewell, powers of the East" (Wright, 2022b).

Last, turn toward the north and say:

"Powers of the North; powers of Air,
Thank you for your presence in our circle today;
For sharing your wisdom and knowledge
Hail and farewell, powers of the North.
Finish the ritual with a final declaration, such as:
The circle is open but never broken!" (Wright, 2022b).

You have officially ended your ritual at this point. Remember that this is just an example of what might occur in a Wiccan ritual and how it can be performed. Wiccan rituals are unique for each person, so there is no pressure to follow exactly what I have shown you. Feel free to tailor it to fit your practice. A lot goes into a singular ritual, but it is worth it in the end because you connect with yourself and nature and make changes. Now that we know of the basis of many Wiccan rituals, it is time to explore the last part of Pillar 5, which is the types of rituals that Wiccans perform.

16

Different Types of Rituals

Every new Wiccan should be aware of a few essential rituals. However, it is impossible to cover them all due to the sheer number and variety. Nevertheless, understanding these fundamentals is key to successful practice. Throughout this chapter, we will talk about four essential rituals all Wiccans need to know, including the centering, cone of power, grounding, and shielding.

Centering

Many Wiccan rituals use energy manipulation, and the start of any energy work is centering. Although there is a common idea of what centering is across the different kinds of Wicca, how someone centers themselves can differ. But to effectively use energy and your magick, you should begin centering yourself. Previous experience with meditation, although it is not needed to learn how to center, can make it much easier because meditation and centering use similar techniques. Practicing meditation outside of rituals can also make it easier to center during a ritual.

To center yourself, find a spot where you will be left undisturbed. If you have children, find a time during the day when you would not be disturbed, such as when they are in school or have a time when they go outside to play. Even if you live alone, make sure there are no disruptions. Turn your cell phone on mute, lock the doors, and turn off the television. You can choose to sit or lie down. Many will opt to sit because lying down might make them too relaxed and lead to them taking a nap. Take deep breaths, in through the nose and out through the mouth. Repeat the process, keeping your breaths even.

Once you have relaxed, it is time to visualize your energy and the energy around you. If you are having difficulty doing this, rub your hands together and hold them close, ensuring they are not touching. At first, you might not feel anything, but you should eventually feel the charge between your palms. This energy should feel like there is some resistance between your hands as you try to bring them back together.

Now that you know what the energy feels like, you can start manipulating it. Focus on the feeling of the energy and then visualize it moving and expanding. It will take some time to master centering, but once you do, you should be able to manipulate energy so that it bends to your will. Centering is not about producing new energy but harnessing what you already have. Visualize bringing your energy forward and forming a ball. Repeat this process to get yourself more familiar with the process. As you continue to practice, it will become more natural, and you can manipulate your energy better.

Cone of Power

The cone of power ritual is all about gathering and directing energy and magick. Both coven and solitary witches can perform this ritual. Naturally, covens produce more power and energy as several witches come together. Meanwhile, a solitary witch can also perform this ritual but would not experience as much energy increase. The cone of power ritual is primarily used as an energy-boosting ritual which allows for spells and other rituals to be more powerful as energy is gathered and released. One of the primary reasons why it is visualized as a cone is that it aligns with the body's chakras. The root chakra, located at the base of our spines, is believed to be the base of the cone, which then tapers as chakras move upwards toward the head. There are various names that someone might use for the rituals, and they might also imagine it as a different shape. But what is important to remember is that many Wiccans use this ritual daily. First, let us discuss how this ritual would be performed with a group.

A magick circle would be cast, and the members who were partaking in the ritual would be inside the circle. The people inside will form a circle, creating the base of the cone of power. Depending on the coven, the witches might join hands, or they might visualize the energy rising from each person, forming a cone. Likewise, the witches inside the circle will chant and sing; as they do this, their power will rise and form a cone of power above them. And based on the coven and the magickal systems being explored, the energy gathered might expand past the cone's apex and float into the world. After enough power has been collected, the coven's leader will complete the ritual, sending the energy toward the group's magickal purpose, including protection and healing. The rest of the ritual would continue, as discussed in the previous chapter.

As we have learned, covens are not nearly as popular as they were at the beginning of Wicca, with most Wiccans nowadays practicing solitarily. Depending on the Wiccan you ask, some say that an individual cannot raise a cone of power by themselves, while others say they can. The process can be done the same way a group would, but only one person exists. How one accumulates enough energy to form a cone can differ depending on the person, with some methods working better than others. Some methods for gathering energy include chanting, singing, drumming, and physical exercise.

Grounding

Connecting with the earth through grounding helps access its healing power and ease anxiety and stress. This method allows you to release energy while drawing upon the earth's power without depleting your own. Earthing helps you, in a sense, recharge your batteries so you have more energy to handle any stressful situations that may come your way. Many natural magick users use grounding because of their inherent connection to the earth.

To ground yourself, sit or lay down with your palms face down. Grounding yourself outside is easier because it allows you to connect with nature physically. You do not need to go into the forest or anything, just into your yard or park. However, if you do not have a safe space in nature to do this process, then doing it inside will be alright. You can either have your eyes closed or open. Imagine your energy traveling through your body, your hands, and then down into the earth. You can also imagine your power traveling from the base of your head, down your spine, and deep into the earth. Where you imagine your energy traveling from will be rooted to where you think it originates. If you think it comes from your head, imagine traveling from there. Or if you feel it in your gut, imagine it traveling from there, into your hands, and then into the ground.

Expelling your energy into the air can help you to find balance and ground your energies. But you need to be cautious and remember that you will not be able to draw onto this magick like you would from grounding it into the earth. Also, discharging magick into the air allows other people to absorb it, which could leave them in a similar position as you are. If you cannot get onto the ground easily, you can also practice grounding by having your bare feet touch the floor or ground and imagine your energy down your body, into your feet, and then into the ground.

Sometimes this is not enough, especially when you first start practicing Wicca. You can try grounding with something tangible, including crystals, phrases, and pots of dirt. As a Wiccan, you likely already have a crystal that you have connected to. When feeling overwhelmed, stressed, or anxious, hold onto your crystal and let it absorb your energy. Create a phrase, simple or complex, that you will say when imagining your energy leaving the body. This can be a great way to finalize the process. Lastly, you can keep a pot of dirt close by, and when you need to expel some energy, place your hands in the soil and feel your energy transferring to it.

Shielding

Shielding is the last of the essential rituals that all Wiccans need to know, as it protects against mental, magickal, and psychic attacks. Likewise, it creates an energy barrier around yourself that others cannot penetrate. However, you can also push magick and energy outside of the barrier. The shielding process is very similar to grounding, but instead of pushing energy outside your body, you will envelop your body with energy. Focus on the ball of energy you form when centering and imagine it expanding around yourself.

Visualize your shield as being reflective. This will repel negative energy and influence back to the person who sent it. Your shield can also be similar to a tinted window, as it will let good things in and keep harmful things out. Shielding techniques can be essential if you are affected by other people's emotions or if you find interacting with specific people exhausting.

These are four essential rituals that all Wiccans need to know when it comes to practicing Wicca appropriately. And now that you have learned them, you have reached the end of this book and know the five pillars essential for Wicca. Before we part ways entirely and you start your Wiccan journey, let us recap what we have learned throughout this book.

Conclusion

When you started exploring Wicca, you might have had a rough time. You might still be going through troubled times, questioning how to connect with yourself and the world more. Stress and anxiety are normal, but Wicca, its practices, and beliefs can all help you get through these challenging times. In the modern day, it has become much harder to connect with oneself, others, and nature as we become more enthralled with technology, but Wicca can help you to connect with yourself, nature, and the divine.

Throughout this book, we learned about the five pillars of Wicca, which are essential for learning and practicing Wicca, and these include the following:

1. **Foundation:** the history and origins of Wicca and Wicca in the present day.
2. **Beliefs:** the deities of Wicca, including the Triple Goddess and the Horned God, the importance of the elements, ethics, holidays, birth, marriage, and death rites.
3. **Practice:** the many different types of Wicca and how to get initiated.
4. **Magick:** natural, ceremonial, and celestial magick.
5. **Rituals:** what is needed for a ritual, how a typical one is performed, and some essential rituals to know.

You have learned how varied and multifaceted Wicca is. It can fit into any lifestyle and help you to align yourself with nature and the universe. The rituals, celebrations, and many Wiccan techniques, such as grounding and centering, can help with self-development and better coping with stress and anxiety. These are essential things to know about Wicca.

Learning about the five pillars of Wicca and starting to practice the Wiccan practices you connect with helps you to harness your intuition and awaken the divine magick inside yourself. Remember that we are all part of the earth, and it is about opening yourself up to the divine to connect with the earth on a deeper level.

Now you have all the information you need to start practicing Wicca and connecting with yourself. I have given you all the tools and information you need, and now it is time for you to take the next step. I know it can be scary to try something new and connect with yourself, but it is time to make positive changes in your life. So, get out there, start putting energy into the world, and rekindle your relationship with yourself!

Glossary

Augury Witches: Wiccans and witches that use their abilities to decipher omens, typically from the behavior of animals.

Beltane: Occurs on April 30th and May 1st and celebrates light, fertility, and the coming of summer. This celebration represents the continued waking up of the earth as more light is brought from the sun. A young girl is often picked to become the May Queen, a stand-in for the Celtic fertility goddess Flora.

Celestial Magick: Magick focused on interactions with the gods in hopes of making earthly changes.

Ceremonial Magick: Magick used to summon gods, goddesses, deities, and spirits. Contains rituals, including banishing, purification, consecration, invocation, evocation, eucharist, and divination.

Cosmic Witches: Wiccans and witches that specialize in astronomy, astrology, and reading the stars. Use spells and moon cycles to protect celestial events and use birth charts and star signs in their practice.

Coven: A group of witches that practice Wicca together, including performing rituals, attending sabbats, esbats, and training.

Coven-Based Witches: witches that practice within a coven.

Crossing the Bridge: The ritual performed during the funeral of a Wiccan. Depending on the Wiccan type you are, how this ritual is performed will differ, but they all honor death. Spiral dances, which represent the cycle of life, are across-the-board.

Eclectic Witches: Are individuals who practice Wicca and identify as witches but adopt other non-Pagan beliefs, philosophies, and practices.

Esbat: Celebrations and festivals that occur during the full moon. These celebrations are not as big as sabbats, and although gods and goddesses are still honored, they do not play a big part. In one year, there are 13 full moons in which the Wiccans will practice.

Gray Witches: Witches that practice white and dark magick, often seeking justice for wrongdoings and redirecting dark magick to appropriate places.

Green Witches: Witches that specialize in healing, nurturing, and nature. They use plants and flowers to make herbal preparations.

Green Witches: Wiccans that specialize in nature, nurturing, and healing. Their tools, rituals, and power are all connected to nature.

Handfasting: The marriage ceremonies that Wiccans have. It is not a Wiccan invention, as it has existed for thousands of years. How the ceremony is performed will differ depending on the person. Still, the primary aspect of tying the couple's hands with colorful ribbons, different fabrics, and cords is always performed. The duration of how long they are tied will vary depending on the people. Handfasting does not equate to legal marriage.

Handparting: The separation or divorce ritual occurs when a married couple no longer wants to be together. Wiccans do not punish divorce; they perform these ceremonies to cut spiritual and symbolic ties. These rituals are supposed to promote continued respect between the partners.

Hearth Witches: Witches are similar to green and kitchen markers, but their practices are centered around the entire house, where they perform protection rituals, herbalism, cleansing, and candle magick.

Hedge Witches: Similar to green witches. However, they do not bind themselves only to the practices of Wicca. Their magick allows them to connect with the elements and create herbal remedies.

Hereditary Witches: Witches born into their powers, typical of later-generation Wiccans.

Horned God: The central male deity of Wicca, who is depicted as a male with horns or antlers or a figure with a male body, but the head of a horned animal. He represents Wicca's male aspects and is the Triple Goddess's consort. He is also a dualistic god, representing two aspects: day and night, light and dark, summer and winter, and life and death. He is associated with the life cycle, hunting, nature, sexuality, and the wilderness.

Imbolc: Is the midpoint celebration between winter and spring and occurs on February 1st and 2nd. This festival celebrates purification and rebirth. Fertility is a big focus of this celebration, as the name Imbolc means in the belly.

Kitchen Witches: Witches that focus their abilities in the kitchen and use herbs in their baking and cooking to extract their medicinal properties.

Litha: Is the celebration of the Summer Solstice and the year's longest day. Celebrations occur between June 20 to 22. As the spirit and human worlds are fully awakened at this time, protection rituals are very commonly used as dark spirits become more powerful.

Lughnasadh: Is the midpoint celebration between summer and fall, occurring on August 1st. The first harvested fruits and vegetables are offered to the Horned God and the Triple Goddess. The Horned God's annual death is known to be approaching, and he is to return to the underworld and Summerland.

Mabon: The celebration of the Autumn Equinox and occurs between September 20-23. This celebration marks the descent of the Horned God into the underworld, where he would not return until after Yule. The second harvest occurs at this time in preparation for winter. This celebration emphasizes reflecting and giving thanks as the soil begins to die in the coming winter months.

Natural Magick: Uses various plants, earthen materials, crystals, alchemy, botany, chemistry, and astronomy.

Ostara: The celebration of the Spring Equinox and occurs between March 20-23. Hope, birth, and fertility are essential to this celebration. The Triple Goddess is said to have become impregnated by the Horned God during this time. Older Pagan generations kept their celebration during this time secret.

Rite of Dedication: A ritual to declare someone's interest in joining a coven. They can start to train with a coven after this rite.

Rite of Passage: A ritual that fully introduces a Wiccan into a coven. Often Wiccans will need to perform various tasks during this rite, typically occurring a year after the rite of dedication.

Sabbat: Seasonal celebrations occur at the turn of the season and in the middle of each season. The eight, or greater, sabbats are depicted on the Wheel of the Year. Usually, witches celebrate Sabbats in a coven and by those practicing solitarily. Solitary witches that know each other will often come together to celebrate the sabbats. The sabbats represent the cyclical nature of life and the seasons. They focus on reflecting on the past and looking toward the future.

Samhain: Celebrated on October 31st and marks the beginning of the Wiccan year. The name means summer's end, and the veil between the mortal and spirit worlds is the thinnest during this time. The transition from summer to fall signifies the end of the light season and the beginning of the dark season. Bonfires are essential for this celebration to mark the continued perseverance of light through the dark season.

Secular Witches: Wiccans and witches that do not equate their powers to religion or spirituality. They do not follow the rules or morals of Wicca and sometimes do not identify as Wiccan.

Self-Dedication: A non-mandatory ritual that solitary Wiccans can perform to dedicate themselves to Wicca, its beliefs, and practices.

Solitary Witches: Wiccans that practice by themselves and without a coven. This is the most common way that Wicca is practiced today.

The Rule of Three: A tenet that many Wiccans follow, which says that what you put into the world will return to you three times. Some interpret this rule as meaning energy will return to them in the form of lessons, often in threes. This pertains to both good and bad energy.

The Wheel of the Year: Is a symbol used to show the eight great sabbats and the 13 esbats celebrated throughout one year. The

Wheel of the Year originated thousands of years before the creation of Wicca and was used by Celts.

Triple Goddess: Also known as a Moon Goddess, the primary female deity of Wicca. She represents the magick number three and triunity. She often represents the female life cycle (maiden, mother, and crone) along with the three realms of the world (heaven, earth, and the underworld). She represented the feminine side of Wicca and became a figure for feminism in Wiccan females because she was a symbol of comfort and liberation.

Wicca: One of the largest neo or modern Pagan religions practiced today. It emerged in the 1960s and was created by Gerald Gardner, credited because of his influence on a coven of witches known as the New Forest Group. Gardner's original writings and practices are now known as Gardnerian Wicca. Wicca, as a religion, has no strict rules and individual covens, and people have created their rituals and theories based on the writings of Gardner.

Wiccans: Followers of the Wicca practices and beliefs and identify themselves as witches.

Wiccan Rede: A poem or speech that outlines the moral standards of Wicca and other Pagan religions. It first started as one line: "An ye harm none, do what ye will" (Wikipedia, 2022a). This was later expanded to be much longer. It is fundamentally the golden rule of Wicca and is interpreted by many to mean: do good to others and yourself.

Wiccaning: The birth rite or welcoming ceremony to those looking to be introduced into the Wiccan's spiritual community. This is not a rite that then makes you practice Wicca but is welcoming you to the community. Many Wiccans will hold this rite for their children, but this does not mean they have to partake in Wiccan practices. Wiccaning is often considered to be the Wiccan version of baptism.

Yule: Also known as the Winter Solstice, it celebrates the shortest day of the year with celebrations between December 20 to 25. Although winter is sometimes associated with death, Yule marks renewing the life cycle as the Horned God returns from the underworld and the days become longer. Evergreens are decorated in honor of the god, and gifts are left out for him. Bonfires and the burning of the yule log also occurs.

References

A list of herbs and their magickal uses. (n.d.).Spiral Rain. https://spiralrain.ca/pages/a-list-of-herbs-and-their-magickal-uses

Alexander B. & Norbeck, E. (2020, November 10). Rite of passage. In *Encyclopædia Britannica.* https://www.britannica.com/topic/rite-of-passage/Life-cycle-ceremonies

Augury. (2023, January 6). Wikipedia. https://en.wikipedia.org/wiki/Augury

Ball, P. (2020). *Natural magick: Spells, enchantments, and personal growth* (pp. 282–290). Arcturus.

Beyer, C. (2019, June 5). *What to know about the five classical elements.* Learn Religions. https://www.learnreligions.com/elemental-symbols-4122788

Ceremonial magick. (2022, December 19). Wikipedia. https://en.wikipedia.org/wiki/Ceremonial_magick

Ceridwen. (2019, March 8). *Elemental magick for beginners: Basic principles.* Craft of Wicca. https://craftofwicca.com/elemental-magick-for-beginners/

Classical element. (n.d.). Chemeurope. https://www.chemeurope.com/en/encyclopedia/Classical_element.html#Neo-Paganism

Eclectic paganism. (2021, July 3). Wikipedia. https://en.wikipedia.org/wiki/Eclectic_Paganism

Esbat. (2022, December). Encyclopedia. https://www.encyclopedia.com/science/encyclopedias-almanacs-transcripts-and-maps/esbat

Horned god. (2022, November 14). Wikipedia. https://en.wikipedia.org/wiki/Horned_God

How to cast a wicca ritual magick circle. (2021). The Not so Innocents Abroad. https://www.thenotsoinnocentsabroad.com/blog/how-to-cast-a-wicca-ritual-magick-circle

Lewis, I. M. & Russel, J. B. (2022, October 21) *Witchcraft: The witch hunts.* (2019). In Encyclopædia Britannica. https://www.britannica.com/topic/witchcraft/The-witch-hunts

Magickal tools in wicca. (2022, November 29). Wikipedia. https://en.wikipedia.org/wiki/Magickal_tools_in_Wicca#Cauldron

Mark, J. (2019, January 28). *Wheel of the year.* World History Encyclopedia. https://www.worldhistory.org/Wheel_of_the_Year/

Patterson, R. (2020, February 14). *The art of ritual: Calling the quarters.* Beneath the Moon. https://www.patheos.com/blogs/beneaththemoon/2020/02/the-art-of-ritual-calling-the-quarters/

Rabu. (2022, October 19). *Apparently, there are different types of witches.* CXO Media. https://www.cxomedia.id/art-and-culture/20221019175249-24-176660/apparently-there-are-different-types-of-witches

Rekstis, E. (2022, January 21). *Healing crystals 101.* Healthline. https://www.healthline.com/health/mental-health/guide-to-healing-crystals

Rule of three (Wicca). (2023, January 2). Wikipedia. https://en.wikipedia.org/wiki/Rule_of_Three_(Wicca)

Shade, P. (2022, October 28). *The supernatural side of plants.* Cornell Botanic Gardens. https://cornellbotanicgardens.org/the-supernatural-side-of-plants-2/

Smith, D. (2016, March 26). *Looking into habits of effective wiccans.* Dummies. https://www.dummies.com/article/body-mind-spirit/religion-spirituality/wicca/looking-into-habits-of-effective-wiccans-201046/

Term: Crossing the bridge. (n.d.) Llewellyn Worldwide. https://www.llewellyn.com/encyclopedia/term/Crossing+the+Bridge

The art of handfasting. (2019, November 19). The Celebrant Directory. https://www.thecelebrantdirectory.com/art-of-handfasting/

The Editors of Encyclopedia Britannica. (2022, December 23). *Reincarnation.* Encyclopædia Britannica. https://www.britannica.com/topic/reincarnation

The wiccan altar: The tools of wiccan ritual. (n.d.). Wicca Living. https://wiccaliving.com/wiccan-altar/

The wiccan rede. (n.d.). Web.mit.edu. https://web.mit.edu/pipa/www/rede.html

Tomekeeper. (n.d.). *Celestial magick.* Luna's Grimoire. https://www.lunasgrimoire.com/celestial-magick/

Triple goddess. (2022, December 20). Encyclopedia. https://www.encyclopedia.com/religion/legal-and-political-magazines/triple-goddess

Triple goddess (neopaganism). (2023, January 9). Wikipedia. https://en.wikipedia.org/wiki/Triple_Goddess_(Neopaganism)#-Contemporary_beliefs_and_practices

Ward, K. (2022, August 26). *FYI: There are many types of witches.* Cosmopolitan. https://www.cosmopolitan.com/lifestyle/a37681530/types-of-witches/

White, E. D. (2022, September 2). Wicca. In *Encyclopædia Britannica.* https://www.britannica.com/topic/Wicca

Wicca. (2023, January 9). Wikipedia. https://en.wikipedia.org/wiki/Wicca#Five_elements

Wicca clothing and ritual attire. (n.d.). Wicca Living. https://wiccaliving.com/wiccan-clothing-ritual-attire/

Wicca manual. (n.d.). Federal Bureau of Prisons. https://www.bop.gov/foia/docs/wiccamanual.pdf

Wiccan cakes and ale ceremony. (n.d.). Wicca Living. https://wiccaliving.com/cakes-ale-ceremony/

Wiccan handparting. (n.d.). Beliefnet. https://www.beliefnet.com/faiths/pagan-and-earth-based/2001/04/wiccan-handparting.aspx

Wiccan rede. (2022, November 14). Wikipedia. https://en.wikipedia.org/wiki/Wiccan_Rede

Wigington, P. (2018a, May 14). *How to sew a simple pagan ritual robe.* Learn Religions. https://www.learnreligions.com/make-a-ritual-robe-2562742

Wigington, P. (2018b, May 21). *Hold a wiccaning ceremony for your baby.* Learn Religions. https://www.learnreligions.com/what-is-a-wiccaning-2562532

Wigington, P. (2018c, December 30). *How to perform a self-dedication ritual.* Learn Religions. https://www.learnreligions.com/self-dedication-ritual-2562868

Wigington, P. (2019a, January 6). *Consecrate your magickal tools.* Learn Religions. https://www.learnreligions.com/consecrate-your-magickal-tools-2562860

Wigington, P. (2019b, February 9). *Celebrate the full moon with an esbat ritual.* Learn Religions. https://www.learnreligions.com/esbat-rite-celebrate-the-full-moon-2562864

Wigington, P. (2019c, March 22). *What is the cone of power in magick?* Learn Religions. https://www.learnreligions.com/the-cone-of-power-2561490

Wigington, P. (2019d, May 8). *The wheel of the year: Celebrating the 8 pagan sabbats.* Learn Religions. https://www.learnreligions.com/eight-pagan-sabbats-2562833

Wigington, P. (2019e, May 9). *14 magickal tools for pagan practice.* Learn Religions. https://www.learnreligions.com/magickal-tools-for-pagan-practice-4064607

Wigington, P. (2019f, June 25). *How to magickally ground, center, and shield.* Learn Religions. https://www.learnreligions.com/grounding-centering-and-shielding-4122187

Wikipedia Contributors. (2022, December 23). *Book of shadows*. Wikipedia. https://en.wikipedia.org/wiki/Book_of_shadows

Wright, M. S. (2022a, August 3). *Beginning wicca: Types of altars*. Exemplore. https://exemplore.com/wicca-witchcraft/Beginning-Wicca-Types-of-Altars

Wright, M. S. (2022b, August 3). *Wicca rituals: A standard ritual opening and closing for beginning wiccans*. Exemplore. https://exemplore.com/wicca-witchcraft/Wicca-Rituals-A-Standard-Ritual-Opening-and-Closing-for-Begining-Wiccans

Printed in Great Britain
by Amazon